Framing Health Care Instruction

Medical Library Association Books

The Medical Library Association (MLA) features books that showcase the expertise of health sciences librarians for other librarians and professionals.

MLA Books are excellent resources for librarians in hospitals, medical research practice, and other settings. These volumes will provide health care professionals and patients with accurate information that can improve outcomes and save lives.

Each book in the series has been overseen editorially since conception by the Medical Library Association Books Panel, composed of MLA members with expertise spanning the breadth of health sciences librarianship.

About the Medical Library Association

Founded in 1898, MLA is a 501(c)(3) nonprofit, educational organization of 3,500 individual and institutional members in the health sciences information field that provides lifelong educational opportunities, supports a knowledge base of health information research, and works with a global network of partners to promote the importance of quality information for improved health to the health care community and the public.

Books in the Series:

The Medical Library Association Guide to Providing Consumer and Patient Health Information, by Michele Spatz
Health Sciences Librarianship, edited by M. Sandra Wood
Curriculum-Based Library Instruction: From Cultivating Faculty Relationships to Assessment, edited by Amy Blevins and Megan Inman
The Small Library Manager's Handbook, by Alice Graves
Mobile Technologies for Every Library, by Ann Whitney Gleason
The Medical Library Association Guide to Answering Questions about the Affordable Care Act, by Emily Vardell
Marketing for Special and Academic Libraries: A Planning and Best Practices Sourcebook, by Patricia Higginbottom and Valerie Gordon

Interprofessional Education and Medical Libraries: Partnering for Success, edited by Mary E. Edwards

Translating Expertise: The Librarian's Role in Translational Research, edited by Marisa L. Conte

Expert Searching in the Google Age, by Terry Ann Jankowski

Digital Rights Management: The Librarian's Guide, edited by Catherine A. Lemmer and Carla P. Wale

The Medical Library Association Guide to Data Management for Librarians, edited by Lisa Federer

Developing Librarian Competencies for the Digital Age, edited by Jeffrey Coghill and Roger Russell

New Methods of Teaching and Learning in Libraries, by Ann Whitney Gleason

Becoming a Powerhouse Librarian: How to Get Things Done Right the First Time, by Jamie Gray

Assembling the Pieces of a Systematic Review: A Guide for Librarians, edited by Margaret J. Foster and Sarah T. Jewell

Information and Innovation: A Natural Combination for Health Sciences Libraries, edited by Jean P. Shipman and Barbara A. Ulmer

The Library Staff Development Handbook: How to Maximize Your Library's Most Important Resource, by Mary Grace Flaherty

Transforming Medical Library Staff for the 21st Century, edited by Melanie J. Norton and Nathan Rupp

Health Sciences Collections Management for the Twenty-First Century, edited by Susan K. Kendall

The Medical Library Association Guide to Developing Consumer Health Collections, by Claire B. Joseph

Searching the Grey Literature: A Handbook for Finding Annual Reports, Working Papers, White Papers, Government Documents, and More, by Sarah Bonato

Transforming Health Sciences Library Spaces, edited by Alanna Campbell

3D Printing in Medical Libraries: A Crash Course in Supporting Innovation in Health Care, by Jennifer Herron

Framing Health Care Instruction: An Information Literacy Handbook for the Health Sciences, edited by Lauren M. Young and Elizabeth G. Hinton

Framing Health Care Instruction

An Information Literacy Handbook for the Health Sciences

Edited by
Lauren M. Young
Elizabeth G. Hinton

ROWMAN & LITTLEFIELD
Lanham • Boulder • New York • London

Published by Rowman & Littlefield
An imprint of The Rowman & Littlefield Publishing Group, Inc.
4501 Forbes Boulevard, Suite 200, Lanham, Maryland 20706
www.rowman.com

6 Tinworth Street, London SE11 5AL

British Library Cataloguing in Publication Information Available

Library of Congress Cataloging-in-Publication Data

Names: Young, Lauren M., 1979–, editor. | Hinton, Elizabeth G., 1981–, editor.
Title: Framing healthcare instruction : an information literacy handbook for the health sciences / edited by Lauren M. Young, Elizabeth G. Hinton.
Description: Lanham : Rowman & Littlefield, [2019] | Series: Medical Library Association book series | Includes bibliographical references and index.
Identifiers: LCCN 2019016000 (print) | LCCN 2019022302 (ebook) | ISBN 9781538118924 (cloth : alk. paper) | ISBN 9781538118931 (pbk. : alk. paper)
Subjects: LCSH: Medical care. | Medical care—Study and teaching. | Medicine—Study and teaching. | Medicine—Vocational guidance.
Classification: LCC R838 .R73 2019 (print) | LCC R838 (ebook) | DDC 610.76—dc23
LC record available at https://lccn.loc.gov/2019016000
LC ebook record available at https://lccn.loc.gov/2019022302

Contents

Preface

Information literacy competencies are crucial for higher education students, including those in the health sciences. The Association for College and Research Libraries (ACRL), a division of the American Library Association, provides guidance on the information literacy skills that students should be acquiring throughout their academic tenure. This resource is being written at a time when instruction librarians from all disciplines are pausing to reflect on the work they do in response to the ACRL's recently implemented theoretical shift in teaching and assessing information literacy proficiencies. The profession previously worked with information literacy competency standards for higher education (commonly referred to as *standards*) since their adoption in 2000. In 2016, the ACRL board of directors rescinded the standards (*ACRL Insider*, 2016); in their place, the board had already established the framework for information literacy for higher education, henceforth referred to as *framework* (Association of College Research Libraries, 2015).

This theoretical shift immediately led to questions regarding if and how librarians should revise their teaching approaches to reflect the framework. Given some time and perspective, we now see many librarians adopting a "both" approach. Many standards-based lessons and teaching strategies naturally carry forward into a framework-based environment. The theoretical scaffolding might look different, but many practical points of application remain the same as we work to prepare students for postgraduate success dependent on efficient, effective information-seeking behaviors.

Health sciences librarians have long been active in this work. It is imperative that we prepare health sciences students with strong information literacy proficiencies as we send them off into careers full of researching, publishing, grant-writing, and seeking authoritative information for their research and for their patients. A review of the literature reveals numerous health sciences librarians focusing on information literacy both conceptually (Knapp & Brower) and also at the undergraduate level (e.g., Franzen & Bannon, Jessy et al., Macy & Coates, Matlin & Lantzy, Zilinski et al., and Van Moorsel), the graduate level (e.g., Brown & Nelson, Kleyman & Tabaei, McClellan et al., Rana, and Swanberg et al.), the postgraduate level (e.g., Hodgens et al. and Schnur et al.), and the professional level (e.g., Ajuwon & Popoola, Hussein et al., Petrak et al., Rosenfeld et al., and Santana Arroyo). So how is this important work continuing in a framework-based environment?

Formatted as a handbook, *Framing Health Care Instruction: An Information Literacy Handbook for the Health Sciences* will analyze bibliographic instruction in the health sciences through the lens of the ACRL Framework. Through descriptive content, case studies, and quick reference ("at a glance") pages, this book will serve three primary purposes:

1. To highlight the important efforts health sciences librarians are undertaking in framework-based information literacy instruction
2. To equip emerging health sciences instruction librarians with theory-aligned practical approaches
3. To inspire seasoned instruction librarians with new approaches and techniques being used by their colleagues.

This resource will take a look at information literacy instruction in progressively higher-stakes health sciences populations (undergraduate, graduate, postgraduate, and professional) in academic and hospital settings. The needs of specific health sciences disciplines will be addressed, as will varying instructional formats and didactic approaches, along with assessment standards relating to information literacy as issued by health sciences accrediting bodies.

REFERENCES

ACRL Insider. (2016). ACRL board takes action on information literacy standards. Retrieved from http://www.acrl.ala.org/acrlinsider/archives/12126

Ajuwon, G. A., & Popoola, S. O. (2015). Influence of motivational factors on utilisation of internet health information resources by resident doctors in Nigeria. *Electronic Library, 33*(1), 103–119.

Association of College Research Libraries. (2015). Framework for information literacy for higher education. Retrieved from http://www.ala.org/acrl/standards/ilframework

Brown, J. F., & Nelson, J. L. (2003). Integration of information literacy into a revised medical school curriculum. *Medical Reference Services Quarterly, 22*(3), 63.

Franzen, S., & Bannon, C. M. (2016). Merging information literacy and evidence-based practice in an undergraduate health sciences curriculum map. *Communications in Information Literacy, 10*(2), 245–263.

Hodgens, C., Sendall, M. C., & Evans, L. (2012). Post-graduate health promotion students assess their information literacy. *Reference Services Review, 40*(3), 408–422.

Hussein, H., Tshuma, N., & Hu, X. (2017). Original research: Health information needs and reliability of sources among nondegree health sciences students: A prerequisite for designing ehealth literacy. *Annals of Global Health, 83*(2), 369–379.

Jessy, A., Bhat, S., & Rao, M. (2016). Assessing the effectiveness of information literacy instruction program: Pre and post evaluation case study. *Library Philosophy and Practice, 1434*. Retrieved from http://digitalcommons.unl.edu/libphilprac/1434/

Kleyman, E. Z., & Tabaei, S. (2012). Information literacy needs in graduate-level health sciences education. *Journal of Physician Assistant Education* (Physician Assistant Education Association), *23*(2), 36–41.

Knapp, M., & Brower, S. (2014). The ACRL Framework for information literacy in higher education: Implications for health sciences librarians. *Medical Reference Services Quarterly, 33*(4), 460–468.

Macy, K. V., & Coates, H. L. (2016). Data information literacy instruction in business and public health. *IFLA Journal, 42*(4), 313–327.

Matlin, T. R., & Lantzy, T. (2017). Maintaining quality while expanding our reach: Using online information literacy tutorials in the sciences and health sciences. *Evidence Based Library and Information Practice, 12*(3), 95–113.

McClellan, S., Detmering, R., Martinez, G., & Johnson, A. M. (2017). Raising the library's impact factor: A case study in scholarly publishing literacy for graduate students. *Portal: Libraries & the Academy, 17*(3), 543–568.

Petrak, J., Markulin, H., & Mati, T. (2008). Information literacy in continuing professional development of medical practitioners: A Croatian example. *Health Information & Libraries Journal, 25*(1), 46–49.

Rana, G. K. (2014). Information empowerment: Predeparture resource training for students in global health. *Journal of the Medical Library Association, 102*(2), 101–104.

Rosenfeld, P., Salazar-Riera, N., & Vieira, D. (2002). Piloting an information literacy program for staff nurses: Lessons learned. *CIN: Computers, Informatics, Nursing, 20*(6), 236–243.

Santana Arroyo, S. (2013). Information literacy for health professionals: Teaching essential information skills with the Big6 information literacy model. *Community & Junior College Libraries, 19*(3–4), 77–91.

Schnur, D., Cheruvanki, B., & Mustafa, R. (2016). The case report: A user-friendly educational tool for psychiatry residency programs. *Academic Psychiatry, 40*(5), 857–858.

Swanberg, S. M., Engwall, K., & Mi, M. (2015). Continuing education for medical students: A library model. *Journal of the Medical Library Association, 103*(4), 203–207.

Van Moorsel, G. (2005). Library-sponsored instruction improves core informatics competencies among allied health students: A research-based case study. *Journal of Allied Health, 34*(3), 145–152.

Zilinski, L. D., Nelson, M. S., & Van Epps, A. S. (2014). Developing professional skills in STEM students: Data information literacy. *Issues in Science and Technology Librarianship, 77*(1). Retrieved from http://dx.doi.org/10.5062/F42V2D2Z

Acknowledgments

We would like to thank our families, as well as the library mentors who have invested in us throughout our careers. Additionally, many thanks go out to our wonderful contributors, who have been so kind to share their efforts in this domain.

Chapter One

Bibliographic Instruction and Accreditation in the Health Sciences

Library instruction. Information literacy instruction. Bibliographic instruction. There are nearly as many names as there are approaches to imparting information literacy skills to higher education students. Information literacy is based on theory but transforms into application in the college classroom. Accordingly, the application—and definition—varies based on the discipline in which it is being taught.

Several of the framework's key components can be identified in varying disciplines' educational accrediting standards. While not an exhaustive list, this is a representative sampling of opportunities for collaboration. Each standard is described below and matched with the corresponding frame or frames.

NURSING (MULTIPLE LEVELS)

It is worth noting that schools of nursing have traditionally maintained strong partnerships with libraries and subject or liaison librarians. This fact is evidenced in the number of nursing case studies representing each of the six frames.

Bachelor of Science in Nursing

Accrediting body: Commission on Collegiate Nursing Education (CCNE)

Essential III: Scholarship for Evidence-Based Practice (Commission on Collegiate Nursing Education, 2013)

1. "Explain the interrelationships among theory, practice, and research.
2. Demonstrate an understanding of the basic elements of the research process and models for applying evidence to clinical practice.
3. Advocate for the protection of human subjects in the conduct of research.
4. Evaluate the credibility of sources of information, including but not limited to databases and Internet resources.
5. Participate in the process of retrieval, appraisal, and synthesis of evidence in collaboration with other members of the healthcare team to improve patient outcomes.
6. Integrate evidence, clinical judgment, interprofessional perspectives, and patient preferences in planning, implementing, and evaluating outcomes of care.
7. Collaborate in the collection, documentation, and dissemination of evidence.
8. Acquire an understanding of the process for how nursing and related healthcare quality and safety measures are developed, validated, and endorsed.
9. Describe mechanisms to resolve identified practice discrepancies between identified standards and practice that may adversely impact patient outcomes."

Related frame(s): Authority Is Constructed and Contextual

Accrediting body: American Association of Colleges of Nursing (AACN)

Essential IV: Information Management and Application of Patient Care Technology (American Association of Colleges of Nursing, 2008)

"Computer and information literacy are crucial to the future of nursing."

Related frame(s): Authority Is Constructed and Contextual, Information Creation as a Process, Information Has Value, Research as Inquiry, Scholarship as Conversation, Searching as Strategic Exploration

Master of Science in Nursing

Accrediting body: American Association of Colleges of Nursing (AACN)

Essential IV: Translating and Integrating Scholarship into Practice (American Association of Colleges of Nursing, 2011)

1. "Integrate theory, evidence, clinical judgment, research, and interprofessional perspectives using translational processes to improve practice and associated health outcomes for patient aggregates.
2. Advocate for the ethical conduct of research and translational scholarship (with particular attention to the protection of the patient as a research participant).
3. Articulate to a variety of audiences the evidence base for practice decisions, including the credibility of sources of information and the relevance to the practice problem confronted.
4. Participate, leading when appropriate, in collaborative teams to improve care outcomes and support policy changes through knowledge generation, knowledge dissemination, and planning and evaluating knowledge implementation.
5. Apply practice guidelines to improve practice and the care environment.
6. Perform rigorous critique of evidence derived from databases to generate meaningful evidence for nursing practice."

Related frame(s): Information Has Value, Research as Inquiry, Scholarship as Conversation, Searching as Strategic Exploration

Doctor of Nursing Practice

Accrediting body: American Association of Colleges of Nursing (AACN)

Essential III: Clinical Scholarship and Analytical Methods for Evidence-Based Practice (American Association of Colleges of Nursing, 2006)

1. Use analytic methods to critically appraise existing literature and other evidence to determine and implement the best evidence for practice.
2. Design and implement processes to evaluate outcomes of practice, practice patterns, and systems of care within a practice setting, health care organization, or community against national benchmarks to determine variances in practice outcomes and population trends.
3. Design, direct, and evaluate quality improvement methodologies to promote safe, timely, effective, efficient, equitable, and patient-centered care.
4. Apply relevant findings to develop practice guidelines and improve practice and the practice environment.
5. Use information technology and research methods appropriately to:

- Collect appropriate and accurate data to generate evidence for nursing practice,
- Inform and guide the design of databases that generate meaningful evidence for nursing practice,
- Analyze data from practice,
- Design evidence-based interventions,
- Predict and analyze outcomes,
- Examine patterns of behavior and outcomes, and
- Identify gaps in evidence for practice.

6. Function as a practice specialist/consultant in collaborative knowledge-generating research.
7. Disseminate findings from evidence-based practice and research to improve healthcare outcomes.

Related frame(s): Authority Is Constructed and Contextual, Information Creation as a Process, Information Has Value, Research as Inquiry, Scholarship as Conversation, Searching as Strategic Exploration

Final Project

"Additional examples of a DNP final product could include manuscripts submitted for publication, systematic review, research utilization project, practice topic dissemination, substantive involvement in a larger endeavor, or other practice project. The theme that links these forms of scholarly experiences is the use of evidence to improve either practice or patient outcomes" (American Association of Colleges of Nursing, 2016).

Related frame(s): Information Creation as a Process, Research as Inquiry, Scholarship as Conversation

In addition to the examples above, the ACRL Health Sciences Interest Group—Information Literacy Standards for Nursing Task Force began collecting research on the specific information literacy needs of nursing students in 2011 and, in spring 2013, submitted "The Information Literacy Competency Standards for Nursing" (Association of College and Research Libraries, 2013). The ACRL board of directors approved the standards in October 2013. These standards are important to mention because they not only address the needs of nursing students of all levels but also the needs of practicing nurses who can apply these skills to continuing education. Each of the five standards is detailed below:

Standard One: The information-literate nurse determines the nature and extent of the information needed.

Standard Two: The information-literate nurse accesses needed information effectively and efficiently.

Standard Three: The information-literate nurse critically evaluates the procured information and its sources and, as a result, decides whether to modify the initial query and/or seek additional sources and whether to develop a new research process.

Standard Four: The information-literate nurse, individually or as a member of a group, uses information effectively to accomplish a specific purpose.

Standard Five: The information-literate nurse understands many of the economic, legal, and social issues surrounding the use of information and accesses and uses information ethically and legally.

DOCTOR OF MEDICINE

In 2017, the Association of Academic Health Sciences Libraries (AAHSL) Competency-Based Medical Education Task Force published a "Health Information Literacy Competencies Map" (Association of Academic Health Sciences Libraries, 2017) for the purposes of aligning the framework with the Association of American Medical Colleges (AAMC), core entrustable professional activities for entering residency; the Liaison Committee on Medical Education (LCME), function and structure of a medical school; and the Accreditation Council for Graduate Medical Education (ACGME), common program requirements. Some of the competency mapping from this effort is referenced below.

Accrediting Body: Liaison Committee on Medical Education (LCME, 2017)

Standard 3.2: Community of Scholars/Research Opportunities. "A medical education program is conducted in an environment that fosters the intellectual challenge and spirit of inquiry appropriate to a community of scholars and provides sufficient opportunities, encouragement, and support for medical student participation in the research and other scholarly activities of its faculty."

Related frame(s): Information Creation as a Process

Standard 4.2: Scholarly Productivity. "The faculty of a medical school demonstrate a commitment to continuing scholarly productivity that is characteristic of an institution of higher learning."

Related frame(s): Scholarship as Conversation

Standard 6.3: Self-Directed and Lifelong Learning. "The faculty of a medical school ensure that the medical curriculum includes self-directed learning experiences and time for independent study to allow medical students to develop the skills of lifelong learning. Self-directed learning involves medical students' self-assessment of learning needs; independent identification, analysis, and synthesis of relevant information; and appraisal of the credibility of information sources."

Related frame(s): Authority Is Constructed and Contextual, Research as Inquiry

Standard 7.3: Scientific Method/Clinical/Translational Research. "The faculty of a medical school ensure that the medical curriculum includes instruction in the scientific method and in the basic scientific and ethical principles of clinical and translational research, including the ways in which such research is conducted, evaluated, explained to patients, and applied to patient care."

Related frame(s): Authority Is Constructed and Contextual, Information Creation as a Process, Research as Inquiry

Standard 7.4: Critical Judgment/Problem-Solving Skills. "The faculty of a medical school ensure that the medical curriculum incorporates the fundamental principles of medicine, provides opportunities for medical students to acquire skills of critical judgment based on evidence and experience, and develops medical students' ability to use those principles and skills effectively in solving problems of health and disease."

Related frame(s): Authority Is Constructed and Contextual, Information Creation as a Process, Research as Inquiry, Scholarship as Conversation

Standard 7.6: Cultural Competence and Health Care Disparities. "The faculty of a medical school ensure that the medical curriculum provides opportunities for medical students to learn to recognize and appropriately address gender and cultural biases in themselves, in others, and in the health care delivery process. The medical curriculum includes instruction regarding the following:

1. The manner in which people of diverse cultures and belief systems perceive health and illness and respond to various symptoms, diseases, and treatments
2. The basic principles of culturally competent health care
3. The recognition and development of solutions for health care disparities

4. The importance of meeting the health care needs of medically underserved populations
5. The development of core professional attributes (e.g., altruism, accountability) needed to provide effective care in a multidimensional and diverse society."

Related frame(s): Information Has Value

DOCTOR OF DENTAL MEDICINE

Accrediting Body: Commission on Dental Accreditation (CODA, 2015)

Standard 2-17: "Graduates must be able to access, critically appraise, apply, and communicate information as it relates to providing evidence-based patient care within the scope of dental therapy practice. Intent: The education program should introduce students to the basic principles of research and its application for patients."

Related frame(s): Information Has Value, Research as Inquiry

DOCTOR OF PHARMACY

Accrediting Body: Accreditation Council for Pharmacy Education (ACPE, 2015)

Standard 21.4: "Librarian expertise access—The college or school has access to librarian resources with the expertise needed to work with students, faculty, and preceptors on effective literature and database search and retrieval strategies."

Related frame(s): Searching as Strategic Exploration

The Center for the Advancement of Pharmacy Education Outcomes also relates to the framework (Medina et al., 2013)

Domain 1—Foundational Knowledge

1.1. Learner (Learner). "Develop, integrate, and apply knowledge from the foundational sciences (i.e., pharmaceutical, social/behavioral/administrative, and clinical sciences) to evaluate the scientific literature, explain drug action, solve therapeutic problems, and advance population health and patient-centered care."

1.1.5. "Critically analyze scientific literature related to drugs and disease to enhance clinical decision making."

1.1.6. "Identify and critically analyze emerging theories, information, and technologies that may impact patient-centered and population-based care."

Related frame(s): Information Has Value, Research as Inquiry

PHYSICAL THERAPY (MULTIPLE LEVELS)

Accrediting Body: Commission on Accreditation in Physical Therapy Education (CAPTE, 2014)

Professional Practice Expectation: Evidence-Based Practice

Standard CC-5.21: "Consistently use information technology to access sources of information to support clinical decisions."

Standard CC-5.22: "Consistently and critically evaluate sources of information related to physical therapist practice, research, and education and apply knowledge from these sources in a scientific manner and to appropriate populations."

Standard CC-5.23: "Consistently integrate the best evidence for practice from sources of information with clinical judgment and patient/client values to determine the best care for a patient/client."

Standard CC-5.24: "Contribute to the evidence for practice by written systematic reviews of evidence or written descriptions of practice."

Standard CC-5.25: "Participate in the design and implementation of patterns of best clinical practice for various populations."

Related frame(s): Authority Is Constructed and Contextual, Information Creation as a Process, Information Has Value, Research as Inquiry, Searching as Strategic Exploration

DOCTOR OF OCCUPATIONAL THERAPY

Accrediting Body: Accreditation Council for Occupational Therapy Education (ACOTE, 2018)

Standard A.6.2: "The curriculum must include course objectives and learning activities demonstrating preparation beyond a generalist level in, but not limited to, practice skills, research skills, administration, professional development, leadership, advocacy, and theory."

Related frame(s): Research as Inquiry, Searching as Strategic Exploration

Standard B.8.2: "Effectively locate, understand, critique, and evaluate information, including the quality of evidence."

Related frame(s): Authority Is Constructed and Contextual, Research as Inquiry, Searching as Strategic Exploration

Standard B.8.3: "Use scholarly literature to make evidence-based decisions."

Related frame(s): Research as Inquiry

Standard B.8.5: "Understand and critique the validity of research studies, including their design (both quantitative and qualitative) and methodology."

Related frame(s): Authority Is Constructed and Contextual, Research as Inquiry

Standard B.8.8: "Write scholarly reports appropriate for presentation or for publication in a peer-reviewed journal. Examples of scholarly reports would include position papers, white papers, and persuasive discussion papers."

DOCTOR OF VETERINARY MEDICINE

Accrediting Body: Association of American Veterinary Medical Colleges (Competency-Based Veterinary Education Entrustable Professional Activities [EPAs]) (AAVMC, 2018)

EPA 5: "Identify questions and information resources. Critique the quality of the evidence and assess the applicability to the clinical situation."

TRANSFORMING ACCREDITATION LANGUAGE INTO A RELATIONSHIP

The discipline-specific information literacies outlined above can serve as a launching point for librarians seeking to begin conversations on their campus about collaborating with teaching faculty. A librarian's knowledge of the accreditation requirements facing teaching faculty will help them establish commonality and a shared fixed point in the curriculum. As the list above is not exhaustive, librarians are encouraged to explore their target programs' web pages for accreditation statements to discern which documentation they should explore for information literacies.

Once the accrediting language has been identified, librarians should determine which frames most closely match the proficiencies listed. An inviting way to begin the collaborative discussion with teaching faculty is to suggest a few frames that you think match the learning outcomes of an assignment with which you both are familiar and allow them to select which frame they would like to focus on in the given lesson. Starting small is advisable—not every assignment has to hit every information literacy proficiency listed in the framework or in the accrediting body's requirements. Over time, as the collaboration strengthens, you should have additional opportunities to weave IL proficiencies into assignments in natural, meaningful ways.

Information literacy will not be the answer to every unrealized student learning outcome or the foundation of every knowledge threshold (for more on threshold concepts, see Meyer & Land, 2003), but every discipline will indeed have information literacies that must be emphasized. The more familiar librarians are with the framework and what an information-literate college student looks like in action, the more opportunities they will have to contribute to the didactic discussions on their campus. There will be natural opportunities over coffee and in committee meetings to highlight information literacies that capture the proficiencies that teaching faculty are desiring to strengthen in their students. Whereas teaching faculty might think of IL as simply citations, librarians can expand the conversation to the concept of the scholarly discourse in a broader sense and how students learn to interact within it. Faculty may automatically think "write a research paper"; librarians can engage students in a discussion of varying publication types and how to best convey their message to their intended audience. The ultimate goal is not to change the learning outcomes on which teaching faculty have long focused but, rather, to partner with them to enhance their approaches in order to lead students to develop deeper critical thinking skills regarding the information that surrounds them.

REFERENCES

Accreditation Council for Occupational Therapy Education. (2018). 2011 Accreditation Council for Occupational Therapy Education (ACOTE) standards and interpretive guide. Retrieved from https://www.aota.org/~/media/Corporate/Files/EducationCareers/Accredit/Standards/2011-Standards-and-Interpretive-Guide.pdf

Accreditation Council for Pharmacy Education. (2015). Accreditation standards and key elements for the professional program in pharmacy leading to the Doctor of Pharmacy degree. Retrieved from https://www.acpe-accredit.org/pdf/Standards2016FINAL.pdf

American Association of Colleges of Nursing. (2006). The essentials of doctoral education for advanced nursing practice. Retrieved from http://www.aacnnursing.org/Portals/42/Publications/DNPEssentials.pdf

———. (2008). The essentials of baccalaureate education for professional nursing practice. Retrieved from http://www.aacnnursing.org/Portals/42/Publications/BaccEssentials08.pdf

———. (2011). The essentials of master's education in nursing. Retrieved from http://www.aacnnursing.org/Portals/42/Publications/MastersEssentials11.pdf

Association of Academic Health Sciences Libraries (AAHSL). (2017). Health information literacy competencies map. Retrieved from https://aahsl.memberclicks.net/assets/05_26_2017_health_information_literacy_competencies_map.pdf

Association of American Veterinary Medical Colleges. (2018). Competency-based veterinary education: Entrustable professional activities. Retrieved from https://www.aavmc.org/assets/site_18/files/cbve/cbve-publication-2-epa.pdf

Association of College and Research Libraries. (2013). Information literacy competency standards for nursing. Retrieved from http://www.ala.org/acrl/standards/nursing

Commission on Accreditation in Physical Therapy Education. (2014). Evaluative criteria PT programs. Retrieved from http://www.capteonline.org/uploadedFiles/CAPTEorg/About_CAPTE/Resources/Accreditation_Handbook/EvaluativeCriteria_PT.pdf

Commission on Collegiate Nursing Education. (2013). Standards for accreditation of baccalaureate and graduate nursing programs. Retrieved from http://www.aacnnursing.org/Portals/42/CCNE/PDF/Standards-Amended-2013.pdf

Commission on Dental Accreditation. (2015). Accreditation standards for dental therapy education programs. Retrieved from http://www.ada.org/~/media/CODA/Files/dt.ashx

Liaison Committee on Medical Education (LCME). (2017, March). Function and structure of a medical school: Standards for accreditation of medical education programs leading to the MD degree. Retrieved from http://lcme.org/wp-content/uploads/filebase/standards/2018-19_Functions_and_Structure_2017-03-22.docx

Medina, M. S., Plaza, C. M., Stowe, C. D., Robinson, E. T., Delander, G., Beck, D. E., Melchert, R. B., Supernaw, R. B., Roche, V. F., Gleason, B. L., et al. (2013). Center for the Advancement of Pharmacy Education 2013 educational outcomes. *American Journal of Pharmaceutical Education, 77*(8), 4.

Meyer, E., & Land, R. (2003). *Threshold concepts and troublesome knowledge: Linkages to ways of thinking and practising within the disciplines.* (Occasional Report 4, ETL Project, Universities of Edinburgh, Coventry and Durham). Retrieved from http://www.leeds.ac.uk/educol/documents/142206.pdf

Chapter Two

Authority in the Health Sciences

Authority is constructed and contextual. This frame is the first that is presented in the Association for College and Research Libraries (ACRL) framework. Though the frames are fluid, overlapping, and not hierarchical in nature, the fact that authority is the first frame discussed in this handbook is meaningful. All disciplines recognize authority, although its sources can vary within different disciplines. Authority can reside in publishing houses, journal titles, authors' names and credentials, specialized databases that have strong trust and name recognition, and the list goes on.

It is important that librarians teaching information literacy to health sciences students introduce the concept of authority so that students have a full grasp when walking out into the work world. They will need to understand the role of authority in publishing, the types of authority that can be found in health sciences resources, and what that means for them when they are trying to evaluate and select the most appropriate resource for their information need.

When consulting the ACRL Framework knowledge practices and dispositions for the authority frame, we find clear hallmarks of students who are proficient in this concept. A lesson plan designed around authority could teach and engage students' grasp of the following concepts:

- Define authority
- Identify various types and levels of authority and health sciences literature
- Consider societal constructs that lead to this authority: What voices emerge? Which voices do not? Why is this?
- Recognize the authority level associated with their information need
- Use appropriate databases and resources to secure information at the authority level required

Specialized content that can accompany a lesson on these topics for the health sciences includes issues like clinical care databases, evidence-based practice (EBP), predatory publishing, and open access initiatives.

One of the first steps in helping students master this frame is establishing a definition of authority. A shared understanding of the terminology that will be used in the lesson is imperative if students are to remain in sync with their instructor.

Authority takes many shapes in our lives, and an effective lesson can begin by drawing correlations to authority in other spheres of our culture. Sometimes we personally exercise authority, and sometimes we fall under authority figures. The same is true in research and academic pursuits. Often, we will consult other authorities in the field, but sometimes we will serve as an authority on a given matter. This can be true even at an undergraduate level; for instance, if students lead their classmates in the lesson for a class period, they become the authority on the topic and need to understand the responsibility that is associated with that designation.

Authority is "a type of influence that is recognized or exerted within a community" (framework). As this frame asserts, "authority is constructed in that various communities may recognize different types of authority" (*Framework* 2015, 12). One of the founding theories behind the ACRL Framework is that of threshold concepts specific to each discipline: once a student has mastered that knowledge, they will never revert back to a state of not knowing or understanding it. Threshold concepts are discipline specific; accordingly, information literacy instructors will benefit from partnering with subject experts to understand what concepts would be central to students' mastery and progression to the next level.

When considering that these concepts are driven by each discipline, it stands to reason that the experts in these concepts are established by each discipline. In the health sciences, there are several distinctions that can render someone an expert and authority on the subject matter. These include subject expertise, societal position, and special experience.

Authority that is based in subject expertise may be the most readily identified and accepted. These experts can be pioneers within a field who established initial principles of understanding upon which others have built or, conversely, visionaries in the field who are imagining what's next. Both can rely upon each other. Here we see overlap between the Authority frame and the Scholarship as Conversation frame, in which researchers are expected to give credit to the work of those who have gone before them.

Societal position is an important basis of authority, although not always initially recognized. Some forms of position are very prominent—institutions of high regard at which experts studied or hold faculty positions, for example. But there are other forms of societal position that can be overlooked. What are the major national powerhouses that produce peer-reviewed literature? Conversely, what voices are left out of the scholarly discourse? Which viewpoints don't make it through peer review and therefore don't enter into the scholarly debate? What are the major science, technology, engineering, and mathematics (STEM) publishers that enjoy numerous submissions and employ high rejection rates, bolstering their authority and reputation?

Finally, we must consider special experience. What sets certain scholars apart? Is it only the things we've already discussed, or are there other attributes that launch someone to the pinnacle of authority? One example of this would be the highly credentialed nature of the health sciences. Those strings of letters behind authors', researchers', and clinicians' names are hard-earned and signify specialized authority within their discipline.

The health sciences feature a unique discussion of authority within the context of this frame. Authority comes in a wide range of levels. Researchers seeking authority and authoritative sources for their research questions will turn to specific sets of sources depending on their precise need. There will be assignments that call for traditional research databases such as Academic Search Premier, JSTOR, ScienceDirect, CINAHL, and MEDLINE. The authority in the articles represented within these databases is similar to those in other disciplines. Experts, often academic, have honed their topic, performed research, and are presenting the results in a peer-reviewed journal. This is the type of research that most students are comfortable with.

Another form of authority resides within a specialized genre of health sciences literature referred to as evidence, which serves as the foundation for evidence-based research. Evidence is evaluated and assigned levels of strength; for example, a systematic review reporting aggregate results from 100 clinical sites has stronger collective evidence than does a single-site study reporting on the same intervention. In a common pyramid-shaped model, evidence ranges from individual-level expertise at the bottom to aggregated results from numerous randomized controlled trials in the form of systematic reviews and/or meta-analyses at the top. More authority rests within resources supported by more independent findings, or evidence, that support the same findings.

Evidence also lives outside these highly structured licensed databases, though. Students must be taught to consult other forms of evidence in order to see the whole picture. If looking to institute a process improvement on the hospital floor on which they are working, they should consult localized evidence sources, for example, hospital guidelines or supervisor guidance. Professional associations provide evidence through policy statements and best practice guidelines. Evidence can also be presented as a dataset from which researchers can extrapolate trends and findings, as found through government resources like the Centers for Disease Control.

Students should learn that all levels of evidence have some amount of value and credence. Though at the bottom of the hierarchical pyramid, the findings of one experienced clinician are still viable and valuable. A lower evidence level does not automatically imply lower value. Many evidence-based assignments call for a blend of evidence levels so that students learn to recognize the value in each evidence format and its application to a well-balanced research paper.

An assignment that helps teach these concepts to students can be quite simple. Having students perform searches using the same or similar keywords in different types of databases allows them to see the variations in each database's holdings, limits, and more. A federated search can lend itself to interprofessional perspectives, which can be valuable for students who will be working in an interprofessional or interdisciplinary capacity. A search in a database such as CINAHL allows students to add specialized health sciences limits including inpatient versus outpatient population, first/any author is a nurse, and target demographics for the patients studied in the research. Turning to databases like JBI and Cochrane allows students to clearly identify hierarchical evidence levels assigned by the databases. Additionally, performing facilitated searching in professional association and governmental data websites allows students to discover resources that can be accessed through the open web. When asked to identify evidence levels for resources found in databases that don't assign levels or found on the open web, students should be instructed to refer to the evidence levels assigned by their professor, as there are variations between evidence hierarchies.

Ultimately, students will be well prepared to engage in the work of determining authority if they are taught to understand what authority looks like within their specific discipline, how it is organized, and where to locate sources to meet their evidence needs. Ideally, students will be introduced to this in their first disciplinary courses as the concepts take time and practice to learn. The hope is that over several years of exposure in an undergraduate or graduate setting, students will feel comfortable engaging in this type of research when they transition to practicing professionals.

Reference: *Framework for Information Literacy for Higher Education.* Chicago: Association of College & Research Libraries, 2015.

AUTHORITY IN ACTION: CASE STUDIES

Evaluating Consumer Health Information Online

Contributor: Chana Kraus-Friedberg, AHIP, MSLS, PhD (Public Health/Pharmacology and Toxicology Librarian, Michigan State University Libraries, Michigan State University)

Frame—Authority Is Constructed and Contextual: Students are asked to explore the editorial and advertising policies of popular consumer health

Authority at a Glance: Quick Tips for Busy Librarians

Q: What is authority?
A: A type of influence recognized or exerted within a community.

Authority Is Constructed and Contextual

Information resources reflect their creators' expertise and credibility, and are evaluated based on the information need and the context in which the information will be used. Authority is constructed in that various communities may recognize different types of authority. It is contextual in that the information need may help to determine the level of authority required.

http://www.ala.org/acrl/standards/ilframework

Types of Authority:

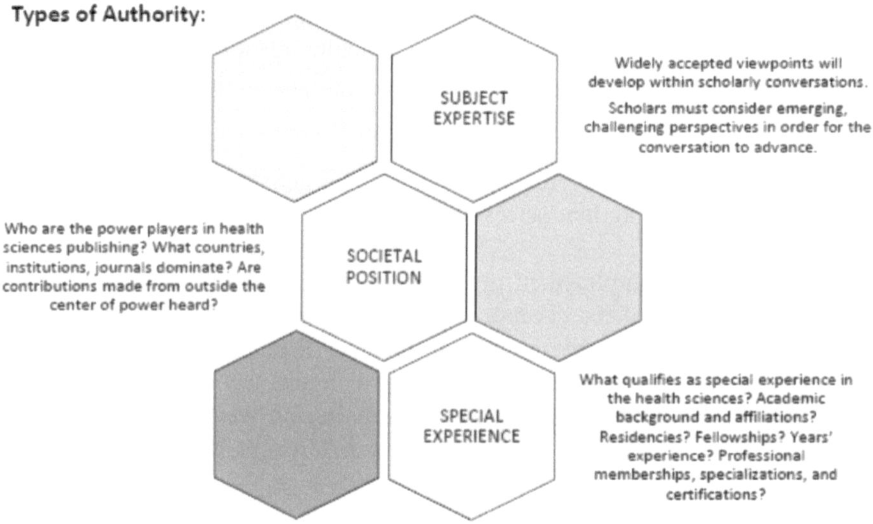

Special considerations for the health sciences:

- ❑ Health sciences disciplines have unique contextual authorities such as evidence-based practice hierarchies and clinical care databases with associated highly authoritative reputations.
- ❑ Health sciences literature is vulnerable to predatory publishing, which renders it critical for scholars to establish authority.

websites. They are then asked to consider what impact these policies may have on the information the website offers, and when this might be important to consider when they are searching for reliable consumer health information.

Other associated frames: Information Creation as a Process; Information Has Value; Searching as Strategic Exploration.

Target Audience: Undergraduate public health students. The lesson may be adapted to other health sciences disciplines, including nursing and allied health.

Setting: Activity accompanying library instruction on evaluating consumer health information for undergraduate students in public health, nursing, or allied health disciplines. The lesson can be used virtually or in person.

Learning Outcomes: At the conclusion of the lesson, students will be able to:

- locate editorial and advertising/product policies on consumer health sites;
- articulate how these policies shape available consumer health information on individual sites and on the web in general; and
- select an appropriate online consumer health resource for a particular information need, taking into account the policies and intended audience of the resource.

Assessment: Student performance on in-class activity (during library session); pre/post-test; student selection/use of resources in their class assignments or papers.

Activity: Best completed in groups, but can be completed individually, either in or outside of the classroom. Target websites can be selected based on the course and available resources. Ideally, different groups of students would be asked to evaluate policies from different websites. Students can then compare their findings in class. Depending on websites selected, students can also be asked to think about the differences between policies of commercial and noncommercial sites. Depending on the length of the class, questions from the "Questions to Consider" section can be selected or omitted.

Evaluating Consumer Health Sites Worksheet

For this exercise, you'll be evaluating a consumer health website that provides information about [health condition or symptom] ____________________. Specifically, you'll be looking at the parts of a website people often don't pay attention to—the editorial policies and advertising policies sections. These sections often give you a lot of information about how content on the site is created and vetted. They are not always easy to find or clearly marked—when in doubt, try searching for an "About Us" link.

Questions to Investigate:

1. Who (or what organization) is providing the information on this website?

2. What criteria are used to determine what topics are covered on the site?
3. Who writes the articles and what are their qualifications?
4. How are articles vetted to make sure that the information they contain is correct?
5. Who does the vetting and what are their qualifications?
6. What happens when incorrect information is published?
7. What criteria are used to determine which advertisers/advertisements should be allowed on the site?
8. How are readers able to tell the difference between ads and informational posts/articles?
9. Does the site link to or cite specific articles or sources? Check a couple of the sources, if you can—do they say what the site claims they say?
10. Are there featured articles or ads that are exempt from the site's policies? Are they clearly marked?
11. Is there a policy dictating how often articles on the site are updated? If so, how often does this happen?

Consider:

- How do you think these factors might impact the kind of information that you would find on this site?
- In what situations would you want to consider these factors when deciding whether the consumer health information on the site is reliable/trustworthy?

Identifying Types of Evidence-Based Nursing Research through Abstract Analysis

Contributor: Kristin E. C. Green, MSILS (Reference and Instruction Librarian, Penn State Scranton)

Frame—Authority Is Constructed and Contextual: By understanding that there is an inherent hierarchy within the types of evidence-based nursing research, students learn that authority is constructed and can be referenced to recommend best practices. By learning about and considering the various types of evidence-based nursing research that constitute the hierarchy, students can place each study within the appropriate context of influence and impact.

Target Audience: Undergraduate nursing students (BSN, RN-BSN).

Setting: This lesson, and corresponding learning activity, occurs during the first of two information literacy sessions for nursing students in the required, writing-intensive, research methods course Principles of Nursing

Research and Evidence-Based Practice. The capstone assignment for this course is a paper in which students research an inquiry formatted in PICO (population, intervention, comparison, outcome). Students are tasked with searching the scholarly literature for the highest level of evidence-based nursing research related to their PICO question that has been accomplished in the field.

Learning Outcomes: Students will be able to:

- understand the hierarchical nature of evidence-based nursing research
- identify different types of evidence-based nursing research

Assessment: The initial assessment for these learning outcomes is conducted through informal group sharing and discussion following the learning activity. Formative assessment of these outcomes continues into the second information literacy session, where students spend time gathering research related to their PICO topics.

The summative assessment for these learning outcomes is the final paper due at the end of the course. Students are asked to include a search methodology section that demonstrates an understanding of the evidence-based nursing research hierarchy. Additionally, students must identify the type of evidence-based nursing research each article exhibits for all the sources referenced in their final papers.

Instruction: Within the nursing curricula prior to this course, students have been exposed to various types of evidence-based nursing research but have not yet been provided a theoretical construct to frame them in. Therefore, this lesson begins with a review of the different types of evidence-based nursing research. Through an informal presentation that welcomes dialogue and inquiry, student misconceptions of the types are clarified.

Instruction continues by introducing students to where these various types of evidence-based nursing research fall within a hierarchy of both filtered and unfiltered information using the Evidence-Based Nursing Pyramid. During this initial part of the lesson, students are acquiring the foundational working knowledge needed for successful development of a key knowledge practice associated with the Authority Is Constructed and Contextual frame; students "define different types of authority" as they learn about the hierarchy and types of evidence-based nursing research (*Framework*, 2015, 12).

Group Activity: Following the instruction of key concepts, students are divided into small groups. Each group is given the same printed packet of six abstracts in which all other bibliographic information is removed. Removal of information must include the articles' titles, as many titles specify a research methodology. Consequently, students are left only with the bare text of the abstracts for their evaluation. Assigning an analysis of abstract text encourages students to "use research tools and indicators of authority," another knowledge practice associated with the Authority Is Constructed and Contextual frame (*Framework*, 2015, 12).

For ease of comparison, the abstracts are all related to one PICO question. This allows students to focus less on the content presented within the abstracts and more on the research methodology employed by the authors. Having the abstracts all relate to a central inquiry also allows the learning activity to more closely mirror what the students will experience as they gather articles related to their PICO questions and typify those sources in their final papers.

In their groups, students try to determine what type of evidence-based nursing research each abstract correlates with by only reading the provided text. Ample time is allotted so groups can reach an internal consensus about each abstract. A class discussion follows covering each abstract in turn, which invariably leads to engaging conversations about authority, scope, and value. Students, representing their group's conclusion, enthusiastically debate when a disagreement arises over the type of evidence-based research an abstract describes. These exchanges are provoked by the intentional exclusion of type, duplication of type, and selection of ambiguous examples, which challenge students to critically think about the constructed authority within evidence-based nursing research.

Beyond the proposed learning outcomes, students learn to appreciate the value of the removed pieces of bibliographic information that may have previously been taken for granted. Students also tend to acknowledge through this activity that reading an abstract may not be sufficient for determining the relevancy of an article to a PICO question. This notion can lead to the awareness that more articles may be gathered and read than will ultimately be used in the final iteration of their research papers.

Reference: *Framework for Information Literacy for Higher Education*. Chicago: Association of College & Research Libraries, 2015.

Interprofessional Group Capstone Poster: Working Collaboratively to Create a Scholarly Product

Contributors: David A. Nolfi, MLS, AHIP (Head, Research Engagement, Health Sciences/STEM Initiatives and Assessment, Gumberg Library, Duquesne University); Rebekah S. Miller, MLIS (Research and Instruction Librarian, Health Sciences Library System, University of Pittsburgh); and Erin Anthony, MLIS (Public Health and Research Support Librarian, John D. Rockefeller Jr. Library, Brown University)

Frame—Authority Is Constructed and Contextual: Students work in interprofessional teams to write a clinical question, distinguish between types of information sources, perform searches in databases, select studies, evaluate study quality, and present results in a poster format. The students also explain the topic's relevance to each of their professions.

Other associated frames: Information Creation as a Process, Information Has Value, Research as Inquiry, Scholarship as Conversation, Searching as Strategic Exploration.

Target Audience: Interprofessional Education (IPE): first-year (pre-clinical) undergraduates in nursing, pharmacy, occupational therapy, physical therapy, physician assistant, speech-language pathology, and health management systems working in teams. This IPE assignment may also be adapted to undergraduate students in other health disciplines.

Setting: This project represents a capstone experience for a one-credit IPE course taught in face-to-face and online formats.

Learning Outcomes: Students work in interprofessional teams to create answerable clinical questions, find appropriate background and foreground sources, evaluate sources, correctly identify study types, and cite sources using a standard style manual. Students work collaboratively to create and present research posters. Students gain an understanding of the importance of IPE and IPP, especially as it relates to health care research, health care ethics, and health equity.

Assessment: Instructors use a rubric to evaluate key elements of the posters including literature searches, results table, discussion of how each health profession addresses the clinical questions, and overall poster design. The rubric includes a 5-point scale to help students understand how to create effective research posters. Students are also evaluated on the group presentation of the poster. Finally, students assess each other's work and key contributions to the group work.

Activity: Research Poster: Students work in interprofessional teams over the duration of a seven-week, one-credit information literacy class to create a culminating, evidence-based final project. The text below provides excerpts from the assignment.

Introduction

The purpose of this group project is to put together what you learned in the course. Through the first six weeks of the course, your group will:

- develop a clinical question based on the PICO format;
- identify background sources;
- learn more about the elements of your clinical question using background sources;
- determine how the clinical question is important to each of the health professions represented by the students in your group;
- find foreground sources that address your clinical question; and

- summarize recommendations about how to best address your clinical question, based on the literature found.

Research Poster

Your group will create and present an electronic poster that summarizes your findings and helps other students learn about your clinical question. Poster presentations are a commonly used way of communicating health sciences research results. Many of you will have the opportunity to present research posters as students (and later as professionals) at health sciences professional conferences.

For this presentation, your audience is other students in the class. Because posters are visual media, include images to help illustrate your project. You should follow the IMRAD structure and include the following:

1. Header
    - Clinical question
    - Group members' names and majors
2. Introduction—the importance of the clinical question in a general context as well as for each health profession represented in your group
3. Methods—Describe the searches that your group conducted for foreground sources, including:
    - Search statements
    - Databases searched
    - Limits/filters you used
4. Results—a table that summarizes your foreground sources. It should include the study, type of evidence, population, intervention, and primary outcome (see table 2.1).
5. Discussion—summarize your recommendations about how the health professionals represented in your group can best address your clinical question.
6. Reference List (on a separate sheet of paper):
    - Your clinical question and group members' names and majors
    - Full APA references for: foreground sources listed in the results table, background sources consulted, and images used on the poster

Make sure to review the sample poster and poster rubric.

Hitting the Reset Button: Using the Unplugging Exercise to Teach How Authority Is Created

Contributor: Amber Loos, MLIS, MPH (Associate Professor and Assessment and User Experience Librarian, Morris Library, Southern Illinois University Carbondale)

Frame—Authority Is Constructed and Contextual: Students will hit the reset button by taking a 24-hour fast from all digital technologies (i.e., smartphone, laptop, television, apps, social media, news sources, etc.). Before they unplug, students will keep a log of the media and information sources they consulted during the prior week. They will evaluate the expertise and credibility of the creators of the media and information they logged. After "the unplugging exercise," students will reflect on their experience, especially as it relates to the lesson goal of understanding how information and media sources can be evaluated for authority.

Table 2.1. Foreground Sources Summary

Study	Type of Evidence	Population	Intervention	Primary Outcome
Allen, W. H., 2015	Cohort Study	Children 2–5 years of age with disease X	Drug A	Reduced duration of symptom Y
Bates, N. W., 2014	Case Study / Series	Children 4–6 years of age with disease X	Drug A combined with Drug B	Reduced frequency of symptom Y
Collins, M. P., 2015	RCT	Child 4–6 years of age with disease X	Drug A compared to placebo	Reduced duration of symptom Y
Dixon, J. P., 2016	Case Control Study	Child 5 years of age with disease X	Drug A	Reduced frequency and duration of symptom Y
Evans, R. L., 2013	Systematic Review	Children 2-6 years of age with disease X	Drug A compared to placebo	Reduced frequency of symptom Y
Farrelly, P. J., 2012	Meta-Analysis	Children of all ages with disease X	Drug A compared to drug B and placebo	Reduced duration of symptom Y
Georgia, 2014	Practice Guideline	Children 2–6 years of age with disease X	Drug A	Reduced duration of symptom Y

Target Audience: This lesson was developed for interprofessional students and can be used across all health sciences disciplines.

Setting: To be used with undergraduate interprofessional students at any level. Students write a self-reflection of their experience of abstaining from all digital technologies for a 24-hour period. This lesson works best over a long weekend or holiday break from classes so that students can more easily refrain from their devices.

Learning Outcomes: Through course lecture, students will become aware of current issues related to media and information sources with a specific focus on bias in information related to health and medical topics (i.e., representation of mental health issues in popular media, how scientific/medical research is translated for the public, debunking health misinformation, etc.). Students will learn to evaluate the authority of the creators of the information they consume and then apply critical thinking skills in order to write a self-reflection on their experience during and after a 24-hour fast from all their digital technologies.

Assessment: Students will complete a reflective paper about their experience with "the unplugging exercise," which will be graded based on the degree to which students sufficiently responded to each of the question prompts.

Activity: The Unplugging Exercise: Students will be given the following activity prompt:

Before "the unplugging exercise," you will keep a log of the information sources and media that you watch, read, listen to, or otherwise consult for a period of 7 days. This log will include a description of what it was (i.e., title and author of the article, video, etc.) as well as information about the expertise and credibility of the creator of it.

During "the unplugging exercise," you will abstain from using all your devices and media for a 24-hour period or longer. You should observe the effects of this exercise on you. After the 24-hour period, you will resume your ordinary behavior with regard to your devices and observe any differences in the types of information and media sources you consume.

The goal of this exercise is to help you notice when, how, and why you consume information and media sources and how you evaluate if it is from a credible source. Also, pay attention to the impulses and feelings that arise in response to being unplugged and summarize your observations.

Please write at least five complete sentences for each of the following questions. Also include a short introduction and conclusion to your reflection paper, for a total of two or three double-spaced pages.

Questions

1. How did being unplugged affect you mentally, emotionally, physically or otherwise? Did you feel much of a desire to seek out information or media during this time?
2. After the 24-hour period, what sources of information and media did you find yourself consuming? Are you able to more easily evaluate the credibility of the sources?
3. What do these patterns suggest about how to use digital technologies in ways that promote credible information from authoritative sources rather than biased sources?

Navigating Veterinary Information as an Independent Researcher

Contributors: Kelly A. Johnson, MS, DVM, MLIS (Veterinary Outreach and Information Resources Librarian, Flower-Sprecher Veterinary Library, Cornell College of Veterinary Medicine); and Erin R. B. Eldermire, MLS (Head, Flower-Sprecher Veterinary Library, Cornell College of Veterinary Medicine)

Frame—Authority Is Constructed and Contextual: Students are tasked with locating and evaluating sources for different stages of an in-class research scenario, recognizing why and how a source's reliability is dependent on information needs.

Target Audience: First-year veterinary students.

Setting: To be used in an interactive manner with first-year graduate veterinary students to inform their approach to a problem-based curriculum. These materials are designed to be delivered in sequential order. For example, an in-class slide presentation can be created to consecutively deliver each concept.

Learning Outcomes: Students will be able to:

1. recognize when information is needed and ask a focused question;
2. locate the most relevant information to answer the question;
3. select the most authoritative sources for each stage of their research, recognizing that a source's reliability is dependent on the specific need or question; and
4. systematically evaluate the information/evidence as it pertains to the need or question.

Assessment: Learning tools can be incorporated to accommodate these exercises for small or large groups. For small groups (less than or equal to 40 students), students can be arranged into groups of three or four and can be given time to discuss each step, then report out to the class for a general discussion before moving on to the next element. This enables instructors to give immediate feedback for all to hear and incorporate. For large groups, software such as Poll Everywhere (https://www.polleverywhere.com/) can be incorporated to generate real-time assessment of student understanding and discussion.

Activity:

Signalment: Hoboken is a 4-year-old spayed female domestic short-haired cat who has been vomiting and lethargic for 4 days. One of the diagnostic tests you run is abdominal radiographs. You need to evaluate the radiograph films as you begin to create your differential list.

To build a constructive search, you need to develop specific, closed-ended questions. For example, asking "How do I evaluate this radiograph?" is too broad and open-ended.

Constructing Closed-Ended Questions

Is the following a closed-ended, searchable question? Why or why not?

"What is abnormal about this radiograph?"

The following is an example of a precise, searchable, and closed-ended question:

"What anatomical structures can be identified on abdominal radiographs?"

What are two or three other precise, searchable, and closed-ended questions instead of the following question?

"What is abnormal about this radiograph?"

Is the following a closed-ended, searchable question? Why or why not?

"What does a normal abdominal radiograph look like?"

Locating and Acquiring Information

Once you've identified precise, closed-ended questions, you need to select appropriate sources to search for your answers.

Are peer-reviewed journals a good source for information about what a normal abdominal radiograph looks like? Why or why not? List an additional two or three appropriate sources.

Another diagnostic test you run is a blood chemistry panel. Would the best resource options differ from those used to address your earlier questions about radiographs? Where would you look to identify normal blood value ranges?

Systematically Evaluating Information

To analyze the blood panel results, construct this closed-ended question: *"What are normal blood chemistry panel ranges for a domestic short-haired cat?"* To answer this question, you search the web and find a blog post from around a year ago, authored by a veterinary technician. When describing a case she had seen in the clinic that day, she included the cat's chemistry profile values as well as normal ranges for reference.

Would you trust the ranges on her blog post as definitively normal? Why or why not?

One way to evaluate the quality of information is to use the CRAAP test (Blakeslee, 2004):

C (Currency)

- When was the information published?
- Has it been revised or updated?
- Is the information current for your topic?

R (Relevance)

- Does the information relate to your topic or question?
- Who is the intended audience?
- Is the information written at an appropriate level?
- Have you looked at multiple sources?
- Would you be comfortable citing this source?

A (Authority)

- Who is the author, publisher, or sponsor?
- What are the author's credentials?
- Is the author qualified?
- Is there contact information?
- What can you learn from the URL (.edu, .gov, .com, .org)?

A (Accuracy)

- Where is the information from?
- Is it supported by evidence?

- Can you verify the information in another source?
- Is the language or tone unbiased?
- Are there errors in spelling or grammar?

P (Purpose)

- What is the purpose of the information (to sell, teach, inform, entertain)?
- Does the author or sponsor make their intentions or purpose clear?
- Is the information fact, opinion, or propaganda?
- Does the point of view seem objective or impartial?

If the blog post were from 10 years ago, would you trust it any more or less? Why?

You have diagnosed your patient with a uterine infection. To treat her, you want to prescribe an antibiotic before you perform surgery to remove the infected tissue. When searching for the most appropriate antibiotic to prescribe, you find information on a drug vendor's website that was posted five years ago describing their antibiotic as the best choice for uterine infections. How does this resource stand up to the CRAAP test? Describe how you evaluate it using each of the five aspects of the CRAAP test:

- Currency
- Relevance
- Authority
- Accuracy
- Purpose

Reference: Blakeslee, Sarah. (2004). The CRAAP test. *LOEX Quarterly, 31*(3). Retrieved from https://commons.emich.edu/loexquarterly/vol31/iss3/4

Assessing the Evidence Together: A Guided EBM Journal Club for Medical Students

Contributors: Emily M. Johnson, MLIS (Assistant Professor and Regional Health Sciences Librarian, Library of the Health Sciences–Peoria, University of Illinois at Chicago); Francis J. McBee-Orzulak, MD (Associate Professor of Clinical Medicine and Program Director Combined Internal Medicine and Pediatrics, University of Illinois College of Medicine at Peoria); and Matthew J. Mischler, MD (Clinical Associate Professor of Internal Medicine and Pediatrics, Associate Program Director Combined Internal Medicine and Pediatrics, and M3 and M4 Clerkship Director, University of Illinois College of Medicine at Peoria)

Frame—Authority Is Constructed and Contextual: Students are asked to form a therapeutic clinical question from their clerkship, translate that question into a search strategy, select an appropriate scholarly article (a randomized control trial [RCT]), and appraise the article's risk of bias, validity, and applicability to that patient.

Other associated frames: Research as Inquiry, Scholarship as Conversation, or Search as Strategic Exploration.

Target Audience: Undergraduate medical students. The lesson may also be adapted to other advanced learners in medicine, such as interns or residents, as well as modified for use in other health sciences disciplines.

Setting: This lesson plan consists of a two-part evidence-based medicine journal club to support third-year students in an internal medicine clerkship.

The first session occurs at the beginning of the clerkship, guiding the students through the search and critical appraisal process based on an example therapeutic patient problem. The session asks students to develop a PICO format question, a guided search exercise on using PubMed (Activity 1) and discussion of the critical appraisal elements for a randomized control trial followed by students applying the principles to the example article.

Students are then expected to submit an assignment on the EBM process (Activity 2), developing their own PICO question, conducting an appropriate search strategy, performing a critical appraisal on that article to evaluate for risk of bias, and demonstrating understanding of basic statistics (absolute and relative risk reduction, number needed to treat, relative risk) (Walsh et al., 2015). The faculty assess the submissions, selecting one student's worksheet to serve as the focus for an applied workshop presentation at the next session.

The second session provides an overview of assignment feedback and the presentation of the selected assignment by the submitting student in a journal club format. The other attending students engage in the critical appraisal of the new article, providing another opportunity for application of the critical appraisal process and engaging in a common presentation format in the medical discipline.

Learning Outcomes

1. Construct a well-built PICO clinical question based on a therapeutic patient problem seen in a clinical setting.
2. Perform a PubMed search using appropriate keywords, medical terminology, and filters based on the chosen PICO question.
3. Select an appropriate randomized control trial based on the PICO question and patient's needs.
4. Critically appraise your randomized control trial based on the risk of bias, validity, and applicability to the patient.

Assessment

Formative: Think-Pair-Share activity to build the PICO question. Instructors and students model the search process and critical appraisal process in a classroom setting.

Summative: Constructive feedback on submitted worksheet of the PICO question formatting, search strategy, and critical appraisal of the selected RCT.

Activity 1: PICO and Search Strategy In-Class Worksheet

Assess the Patient: Clinical Scenario

Ask the Clinical Question: Write a clinical question containing all the components defined in your PICO (see table 2.2).

Acquire Evidence in PubMed: Use Clinical Queries to find quick results for your PICO question. Document your search strategy.

- Use MeSH subject headings and filters to search for journal literature. Document your search strategy.
- Be prepared to report on strengths and weaknesses for each type of search.

Activity 2: Critical Appraisal Worksheet for Submission

Based on Critical Appraisal Questions in the *Users' Guides to the Medical Literature* (Walsh et al., 2015)

Journal Club Worksheet
Therapy Article

1. Clinical Question

    - P(Pt/population)
    - I(Intervention)

Table 2.2. PICO Table

Framework	Self: Response	Team: Response
P		
I		
C		
O		
Question Type		
Study Type		

- C(Comparison)
- O(Outcome)

2. Provide your PubMed search strategy you used to find your article.
3. Why did you select these search terms, and why do you believe the search strategy addresses your clinical question?
4. PubMed Citation
5. Are the results of this therapeutic study *valid*?

   - Was the assignment of patients to treatment randomized? Was allocation concealed?
   - Were patients, clinicians, and study personnel kept "blind" to treatment?
   - Were the groups similar at the start of trial?
   - Were the groups treated equally other than the experimental treatment?
   - Was intention-to-treat analysis performed?
   - Were all subjects properly accounted for and attributed at its conclusion?

6. What are the *results*? (See table 2.3.) What was the treatment effect? (Calculate RRR, ARR, NNT. See table 2.4.) How precise was the estimate of effect (95% CI)?
7. How does this apply to my patient?

   - Can I apply the results to my patients?
   - Were all clinically important outcomes considered?
   - Is the treatment feasible in my setting?
   - Are treatment benefits worth the harms and costs?

Reference: Walsh, M., Perkovic, V., Manns, B., Srinathan, S., Meade, M. O., Devereaux, PJ, & Guyatt, G. (2015). Therapy (randomized trials). In G. Guyatt, D. Rennie, M. O. Meade, & D. J. Cook (Eds.), *Users' Guides to the medical literature: A manual for evidence-based clinical practice* (3rd ed.). New York, NY: McGraw-Hill Education.

Table 2.3. Treatment Outcome

	Outcome Present	Outcome Absent
Treatment	a	b
Placebo	c	d

Table 2.4. Risk Reduction (CER = Controlled Event Rate / EER = Experimental Event Rate)

		Relative Risk Reduction (RRR)	Absolute Risk Reduction (ARR)	Number Needed to Treat (NNT)
CER	EER	CER-EER CER	CER-EER	1/ARR

Chapter Three

Information Creation as a Process

"Information in any format is produced to convey a message and is shared via a selected delivery method. The iterative processes of researching, creating, revising, and disseminating information vary, and the resulting product reflects these differences" (*Framework* 2015, 14). This brief definition from the Association for College and Research Libraries' description of the frame will serve as a guide for our discussion in this introduction and inspires our outline:

- Information comes in multiple formats.
- Information is produced to convey a message.
- Information is shared via a select delivery method.
- Information creation involves the iterative processes of researching, creating, revising, and disseminating information.
- The end product of information creation reflects the differences in the approaches.

INFORMATION COMES IN MULTIPLE FORMATS

Information comes in multiple formats. Academic and professional researchers enjoy a wide variety of avenues in which to publish their findings. With the advent of electronic publishing, the options may seem overwhelming to some novice researchers. They could wonder: What publication type will be the best avenue to share my research with the world? Which will have the greatest impact, and which will reach my intended audience?

Some of the most common forms that health sciences researchers turn to include poster sessions, delivered papers, newsletter and other informal writing opportunities, books and book chapters, and scholarly journals.

A poster session's impact is determined by the given discipline. Typically presented at professional meetings and conferences, these initial research findings are highly valued by some disciplines. They are a common introductory research delivery mechanism for students, with many institutions and associations holding student research days and poster presentation days. Posters are a wonderful choice when the information you are seeking to present has a visual element. Can your findings be best described using a time line? A graph? Images? If you answered yes, a poster might be the best avenue for you. There are varying formats for poster creation—different researchers approach it in different ways. Some create the whole presentation and simply send off for publication, whereas others in the information world allow others to design for them. Researchers even have options when it comes to printing, such as paper-based posters versus cloth-based posters that can be folded into luggage and ironed on-site.

Posters are visually engaging when done well and can create an instant connection between the researcher and the audience. But some types of research don't lend themselves to a poster session. Another format of sharing research directly with your peers is delivering a paper presentation at a conference or a meeting. Papers and posters both go through a peer-review process, by which authors submit proposals in advance of the meeting and a panel blindly evaluates the submissions for appropriateness, quality, and impact. When selected for a paper presentation, the authors should prepare a manuscript that can be shared with the audience attending the paper. Many conferences see researchers developing PowerPoint presentations to create a visual hook and to aid in information retention. The time invested in a paper and its accompanying presentation can be quite high, but in some fields, it is considered a higher-impact publishing option than a poster.

Posters and papers can be stand-alone entities, or they can be starting points for further development of the research and preparation for a scholarly article. In the health sciences, peer-reviewed scholarly journals reign as the publication format with the most impact. Critical to promotion and tenure, peer-reviewed articles serve as a foundation for researchers in health sciences fields. Members of a given discipline can serve on the editorial review board for given journals and will blindly evaluate the article proposals for applicability to the journal, currency, relevancy, interest, quality, and impact. Reviewers provide comments and recommendations to the editor, who then decides whether to invite the author to make the required changes, or to decline the article for publication.

Students and new researchers in the health sciences will need help finding the appropriate journals for article submissions. Bibliographic tools such as Journal Citation Reports and Scopus allow librarians and scholars to identify journals with high impact in their field. With this impact naturally comes authority and respect. An article line on a CV can have varying value depending on the journal of publication. The type of journal article can also be received differently by promotion and tenure committees; for example, a case study in a peer-reviewed journal can have a different value than an empirical research study using a statistical methodology. Researchers need to learn what is valued in their profession in order to succeed. Librarians can support them by helping them identify the available journal and publishing options.

Another form of scholarly writing is more casual in nature and can include writing for newsletters, websites, and professional association sections and interest groups. This type of writing can fall as much under service as it does scholarly publication but helps create a full professional body of work that demonstrates the individual's engagement within their discipline.

INFORMATION IS PRODUCED TO CONVEY A MESSAGE

According to the *American Heritage Dictionary of the English Language*, information can be defined thusly: 1) Knowledge or facts learned, especially about a certain subject or event; and 2) the act of informing or the condition of being informed; communication of knowledge. Rarely do professionals seek to obtain new understanding without plans to apply that new knowledge in a meaningful way. One such meaningful way is to inform their colleagues of new discoveries, insights, and findings on the topic at hand through publication. The previous section details numerous types of information projects health sciences researchers can create, each with unique impact on the scholarly discourse. Further discussion of the impact each can hold will be pursued in the next section: selecting an information delivery method.

INFORMATION IS SHARED VIA A SELECTED DELIVERY METHOD

As previously discussed, information comes in a variety of formats, and the main goal for information is to deliver new knowledge to peers in a given field. When a researcher is selecting which delivery method to use for their information, they must consider the impact that each format will have on the academic community and the existing scholarly discourse.

With options ranging from informal newsletter articles and live presentations at conferences and meetings, to high-quality scholarly works appearing in peer-reviewed journals and books, researchers have numerous options for information delivery. And the decisions don't end there. Once they have selected the medium for their research, they still need to make further selections on how it will be delivered. We live in a world of information duality: information in the health sciences thrives in online formats as well as in print.

Researchers must choose from a number of publishing options, from open access to traditional licensed journal models. Authors also need to remain abreast of guidelines calling for transparency in research findings when funded by tax monies.

There are pitfalls that plague the entire publishing industry, which have particular relevance in an increasingly cutthroat STEM environment. Predatory publishing is a model in which fake publishers create very convincing publisher web pages and advertise open access models in which article authors will shoulder publication fees. But publication doesn't often occur. The scammers pocket the open access fees, and the author is left out of money and with a publication pending that cannot be legitimately published elsewhere; or, authors will balk at the publication fee and ask to remove the article from publication consideration, and the predatory publisher decides to publish anyway. This can be very detrimental to the authors because they not only are associated with a predatory journal but also will have difficulty publishing their findings in a refereed scholarly journal. Researchers in highly competitive fields can be vulnerable to these bad actors as they scramble to be the first to make a claim or share a finding. Pursuing publication through traditional journal routes can take 18 months or longer from article submission to publication, and many highly reputable journals have extremely high rejection rates. With scholarly reputation and often tenure on the line, it's no wonder that anxious scholars could be convinced to take an offer that is ultimately too good to be true.

INFORMATION CREATION INVOLVES THE ITERATIVE PROCESSES OF RESEARCHING, CREATING, REVISING, AND DISSEMINATING INFORMATION

Bloom's Taxonomy is a model that presents a hierarchy of verbs to indicate the level of associated didactic cognitive tasks (Bloom et al., 1956). Information creation employs high-level Bloom's Taxonomy skills such as creating, interpreting information, revising, and disseminating. These skills are complex, and novice researchers will not master them the first time. Repeating these processes will help researchers hone their proficiency at the skills. This difficulty of mastery that lends itself to repetition renders these processes iterative. A process is iterative when through repetition the learner gradually acquires and applies new concepts.

The act of performing research is iterative in that new scholars will become increasingly comfortable and familiar with information sources that contain literature relevant to their discipline. They will learn what keywords elicit the results they are seeking. They will learn the limits that have the most impact on their searching. They will learn Boolean operators that can expand and refine their search results quickly and efficiently. But research is not just the act of locating articles in a database. Research involves a much higher level of critical thinking skills such as reading, interpreting, integrating, and determining if a resource fulfills the researcher's information need. These skills require repeated exposure to scholarly journal articles and other publishing mediums. Students must become familiar with the format of a scholarly article, the jargon and terminology associated with their discipline, and how to determine applicability to their research question. These are all skills that teaching faculty and librarians can both contribute to developing in students.

The act of creation sees a scholar's internalized knowledge develop into something that is shareable with others in their field. For some, it is a skill that comes easily; for others, it is a process that requires much practice and mentoring to see ideas take form on paper. The twin of creation is revision. Every scholar needs to step back and reflect upon what they put on paper. Were the goals met? Did the words convey the spirit of the ideas? Are the correct citations used to show growth in a given discipline? Many elements of a research project are benefited by close revision.

Finally, the dissemination of the research is a highly iterative process. Novice researchers will have questions and uncertainties from the very beginning: How do I pick a journal for submission? How do I know if it's a good one in my field? This is an opportunity for librarians to discuss the means of assessing article, journal, publisher, and even author impact using both licensed and open access tools.

THE END PRODUCT OF INFORMATION CREATION REFLECTS THE DIFFERENCES IN THE APPROACHES

After following the flow of decision making in the publication process, the researcher should have an end product that will reflect their carefully made choices. With information type, audience, and delivery preference in mind, the author can employ research strategies that best emphasize a project's place within the scholarly discourse; creation and revision decisions that best speak to the audience; and dissemination format(s) that will reach the desired audience using the most impactful platforms.

REFERENCES

Framework for Information Literacy for Higher Education. (2015). Chicago: Association for College & Research Libraries.

Information. (2016). In *The American Heritage(R) Dictionary of the English Language* (5th ed.). New York, NY: Houghton Mifflin.

Creation at a Glance: Quick Tips for Busy Librarians

Information Creation as a Process

Information in any format is produced to convey a message and is shared via a selected delivery method. The iterative processes of researching, creating, revising, and disseminating information vary, and the resulting product reflects these differences.

http://www.ala.org/acrl/standards/ilframework

Pedagogical Point: Iteration
A process is iterative when, through repetition, the learner gradually acquires and applies new concepts.

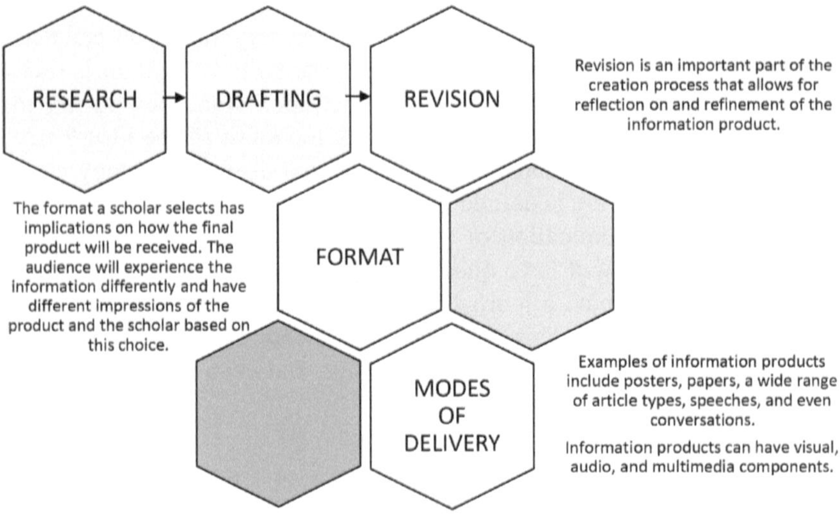

Special considerations for the health sciences:

- ❑ Many health sciences scholars release initial research results in poster and presented paper format, which can be found as grey literature via association websites and journals. Scholars in this field need to recognize the value but also the limitations of varying publication formats.
- ❑ Health sciences journals are increasingly offering multimedia components on their home pages, such as interactive modules, videos, and CME offerings. Scholars should consider how they might cite such a resource before determining to use its information in their research.

FRAMING HEALTHCARE 2

Bloom, B. S., Engelhart, M. D., Furst, E. J., Hill, W. H., & Krathwohl, D. R. (1956). *Taxonomy of educational objectives: The classification of educational goals*. New York, NY: Longmans, Green.

CREATION IN ACTION: CASE STUDIES

Peer-Reviewed Articles and Patient-Care Entries: Process and Purpose

Contributor: Michelle Price, MLS, MA (Outreach and Special Collections Librarian, Liaison to the Wegmans School of Nursing, Lavery Library, St. John Fisher College)

Frame—Information Creation as a Process

Target Audience: Upper-division (300–400 level) undergraduate nursing students. The lesson may also be adapted to other health disciplines that use evidence-based care tools like UpToDate or DynaMed Plus. Applicable to graduate students as well.

Setting: Senior-year undergraduate nursing students who have already received three curriculum-mapped, scaffolded, library instruction sessions. The lesson is currently deployed in a face-to-face classroom, but the activities could be adapted for an online environment.

Learning Outcomes: Students will:

- analyze the process of becoming an author in a traditional peer-review process, and for a patient-care entry;
- contrast the structure, authorship, and evidence base of a scholarly review article and a patient-care entry on the same topic; and
- determine the scope of issues addressed by scholarly articles and patient-care entries.

Assessment: Assessment strategy and desired outcomes such as the following:

- What do I want students to learn? DynaMed Plus is a tool and has limitations like all tools.
- Enduring understanding: Tools are created with an audience and specific purpose in mind.
- Essential Question: Why might a physician/nurse/physician assistant use DynaMed Plus? A scholarly review article?
- What specific knowledge do students need to know? Editorial Process and Authorship Selection.
- How will I know if students have learned? Explain the difference between the peer-review process of DynaMed and the traditional peer-review process of a scholarly journal.
- What indicators will you look for? Compare two entries regarding asthma and pregnancy. Accurately list the selection process of authors and de-

scribe the peer-review process. Description of situations of when to use a patient-care entry or a scholarly peer-reviewed article.

Summative Assessment Example: Collect worksheets and evaluate the following two questions:

1. In what situations would a health care provider use an UpToDate entry? Why?
2. In what situations would a health care provider use scholarly peer-reviewed articles? Why?

The questions assess student learning outcomes directly related to American Association of Colleges of Nursing Essentials of Baccalaureate Education for Professional Nursing Practice:

- 3.2. Demonstrate an understanding of the basic elements of the research process and models for applying evidence to clinical practice.
- 3.4. Evaluate the credibility of sources of information, including but not limited to databases and internet resources.

Rubric: Students receive a point for each question answered, for a total of 2 points (table 3.1).

Activity: The peer-review video is played by the instructor to start the activity. Students then complete questions 1–6 in pairs or small groups. The instructor posts a grid on a dry-erase board and asks for volunteers to put their answers to the questions up on the board. Teacher Prompt: What do you think could be a benefit of entries that are constantly revised? What is a drawback?

After a discussion of the posted answers, the students complete the chart in question 7. The instructor provides direct links to the full text in the classroom worksheet. After completion, the instructor reviews the chart, soliciting verbal answers from students. Teacher Prompt: What are the qualifications or credentials of the authors from both items? What types of sources are listed in the reference list, original articles, review articles, and/or clinical practice guidelines?

Table 3.1. Assessment Rubric

	0	**1**	**2**
Question	Answered None, or Both Answers Incorrect	Answered One, or Only One Correct Answer	Answered Two; Both Answers Correct

The instructor then moves into the last activity, which could be teacher led or student exploration depending on time and instructor preference. Teacher Prompt: What about the structure of a DynaMed entry helps it meet the purpose of helping health care providers find the right information faster? Would DynaMed help answer workforce questions such as risks/benefits of 8-hour versus 12-hour work shifts?

Scholarly Peer-Review Process

http://goo.gl/SfDoqL (3-minute video)

1. Who decides who gets to write an article (be the author of an article)?
2. At what point in the process do peers evaluate content?
3. At what point in the process are revisions made?

DynaMed Process

https://goo.gl/fS6fuL (website)

1. Who decides who gets to write an article (be the author of an article)?
2. At what point in the process do peers evaluate content?
3. At what point in the process are revisions made?
4. Compare and contrast.
5. In what situations would a health care provider use a DynaMed entry? Why? (Please include an example.)
6. In what situations would a health care provider use a scholarly journal article? Why? (Please include an example.) See table 3.2.

Peer Review, Open Access, and Predatory Publishing: Evaluating Sources in Undergraduate Nursing Research

Contributor: Jenessa McElfresh, MLIS, AHIP (Health Sciences Librarian, Clemson University Libraries, Clemson University)

Frame—Information Creation as a Process: Other associated frames: Scholarship as Conversation.

Target Audience: Undergraduate nursing students (RN-BS, BS, Accelerated BS). The lesson can be adapted to other health or life sciences curriculums, including public health sciences, biology, or pre-professional programs in the health sciences.

Setting: Accompanies sophomore- or junior-level undergraduate one-shot library instruction lesson on finding and evaluating nursing research, as part of a course on research in nursing. Students in this course are required to find and critique published research articles individually and in groups.

Learning Outcomes: Students will be able to:

Table 3.2. Resource Comparison

	Asthma Outcomes and Management during Pregnancy: *Chest*	**Asthma during Pregnancy: *DynaMed***
Number of authors/editors		
Length (pages/paragraphs)		
Sections (# and examples)		
Last updated date		
# of references		
Information regarding PEFR (Peak Expiratory Flow Rate)		

- describe the context of peer review in open access and traditional publishing, including the role of predatory publishing,
- discover and compare reputable research articles with articles published in predatory publications found in library databases and other web sources, and
- create criteria that indicate the scholarly trustworthiness of an article and signify appropriate inclusion in undergraduate nursing research.

Assessment: Formative, competency-based assessment at the end of the lesson is suggested to measure the students' success in meeting stated learning outcomes. This can be done using a quick, 5-minute True or False and open-ended quiz using online polling software such as Google Forms or Poll Everywhere.

True or False assessment statement suggestions:

- Peer review is a necessary benchmark to evaluate an article for credibility.
- All open access articles are the result of predatory publishing.
- If it appears in a database, it is a reputable scholarly source.

Open-ended prompt suggestions:

- Why is peer review important in nursing research?
- How do you think this lesson might impact how you find and evaluate articles in the future?
- What tools might you use in the future to evaluate articles for credibility and use in nursing research?

Activity—Scholarly and Predatory Article Investigation Exercise: To be completed in class following librarian-led introduction to publishing models and class discussion on the value of peer review in nursing and health care research. Students work in groups while investigating. Following this exercise, the class comes together to discuss the differences in the articles and works collaboratively to form a list of criteria that make up a valid scholarly source. The articles are selected by the librarian before class and can be tailored to discipline or class material.

Scholarly and Predatory Article Investigation Exercise

With your group, take a close look at the two articles provided. One article is from a reputable scholarly source, and the other is from a predatory publisher.

Using library databases like CINAHL and MEDLINE, scholarly analysis tools like Ulrichsweb and Cabell's Scholarly Analytics, and web tools like Google, appraise the articles according to the criteria listed below.

Once you have answered the following questions, discuss the differences in the articles with your group and what led to your final conclusions.

Article 1

Article Title:
Author(s):
Journal Title:
Volume and Issue:
Year Published:
DOI:
Journal Impact Factor:
Is this article peer reviewed? Y or N / How can you tell?
Were you able to find this article in a library database? Y or N
Were you able to find this article's full text on the web? Y or N
Can you find other articles published in this journal? Y or N
Publisher of Journal:
Does the publisher website look professional? Y or N
Does this journal have an editorial board? Y or N
How long has this journal been published?
Do authors need to pay to publish in this journal? Y or N
How do authors submit manuscripts to this journal?
Do you think this article is reputable or predatory? Y or N
Would you use it in your nursing research paper? Y or N

Article 2

Article Title:

Author(s):
Journal Title:
Volume and Issue:
Year Published:
DOI:
Journal Impact Factor:
Is this article peer reviewed? Y or N / How can you tell?
Were you able to find this article in a library database? Y or N
Were you able to find this article's full text on the web? Y or N
Can you find other articles published in this journal? Y or N
Publisher of Journal:
Does the publisher website look professional? Y or N
Does this journal have an editorial board? Y or N
How long has this journal been published?
Do authors need to pay to publish in this journal? Y or N
How do authors submit manuscripts to this journal?
Do you think this article is reputable or predatory? Y or N
Would you use it in your nursing research paper? Y or N

Introduction to Research Methods in Global Health

Contributor: Kathy Butler, MLS, AHIP (Health Sciences Librarian, George Mason University)

Frame—Information Creation as a Process: Students are introduced to epidemiology as a core research method in public health, and challenged to evaluate the quality of evidence of different methodologies using the Quality of Evidence Pyramid. Other associated frames: Authority Is Constructed and Contextual.

Target Audience: Undergraduate students in public health. The lesson may also be adapted to other health sciences disciplines, including nursing.

Setting: Sophomores enrolled in Introduction to Global Health, either as introductory requirement for a public health major or as part of new core university requirements for developing global citizenship. The description in the course catalog includes the statement "and basic methods used to study global health" (GMU course catalog 2019–2020). The lesson plan can be used in face-to-face classes or as a BlackBoard module.

Learning Outcomes: Students will:

- define epidemiology as a research methodology in public health,
- identify types of research articles used in evidence-based medicine, and
- question the quality of evidence based on methodology.

Assessment: Depending on the size of the class, asking for student responses to questions will guide assessment. The activity will assess how well the concept of quality of evidence is applied to specific articles.

Activity 1

1. Show miasma theory and vibrio cholera and briefly describe history of cholera epidemics in 19th-century London. Identify John Snow as one of the first epidemiologists.
2. Show 7 minutes of video *England: The Broad Street Pump—III: Map of the Blue Death—Extra History*: https://youtu.be/9NVT6iZP2qg.
3. Define epidemiology using the five *W*'s (what, who, where, when, why/how) and three *D*'s (distribution, determinants, disease): https://www.cdc.gov/publichealth101/epidemiology.html.
4. Show two title pages from epidemiological studies. Ask the group the following question: Why are these public health research studies?

    a. Huang, Q., Hu, L., Liao, Q., Xia, J., Wang, Q., & Peng, H. (2017). Spatiotemporal analysis of the malaria epidemic in mainland China, 2004–2014. *American Journal of Tropical Medicine and Hygiene, 97*(2), 504–513. doi:10.4269/ajtmh.16-0711
    b. Mace, K. E., Arguin, P. M., & Tan, K. R. (2018). Malaria surveillance—United States, 2015. *Morbidity and Mortality Weekly Report. Surveillance Summaries* (Washington, DC: 2002), *67*(7), 1–28. doi:10.15585/mmwr.ss6707a1

5. Show study design tree from CEBM (https://www.cebm.net/2014/04/study-designs/). Comment on what kinds of research fit each branch of tree. Where does epidemiology fit?
6. Show quality of evidence pyramid from Ingham-Broomfield, R. (2016). A nurses' guide to the hierarchy of research designs and evidence. *Australian Journal of Advanced Nursing, 33*(3), 38–43. Explain the methodology for each level. Make the point that this is for medicine/health care only; missing methodologies are Qualitative and Mixed Methods research, which are important in other disciplines (history, social sciences).
7. Show titles of articles and abstracts—what kind of study are they according to the pyramid? What level of evidence are they? (Show of hands.)

Activity 2

In groups of four or five, give each group five title pages marked with author name; ask each group to rank the title pages in order of evidence 1=Highest, 5=Lowest. After 5 minutes, each group goes to the whiteboard and ranks articles (using author names) from 1 to 5. Compare the results. How do you know what kind of methodology is used from the title or abstract?

Ask for questions.

"Speed Dating" with Social Work Resources

Contributor: Elena Azadbakht (Health Sciences Librarian, Mathewson-IGT Knowledge Center, University of Nevada, Reno)

Frame—Information Creation as a Process: Students—working in groups of two or three—are provided with several different source types related to a specific topic or problem and are tasked with evaluating these sources. Students must also consider how the sources' content might inform their understanding of the topic or problem. Thus, they become familiar with a variety of different information formats found in the field of social work as well as each format's unique characteristics. Students also gain practice determining if and how a particular source fulfills an information need within a given context. Another associated frame is Authority Is Constructed and Contextual.

Target Audience: Undergraduate social work students. The lesson may also be adapted to other health sciences disciplines, such as public health and kinesiology. This activity may also benefit new graduate students.

Setting: This activity was designed with an upper-level undergraduate social work course in mind. Ideally, the students will have previously attended a library instruction session in which they refined their searching skills and are now ready to focus on appraising sources.

Learning Outcomes: Students will become familiar with several common social work information source types (e.g., peer-reviewed journal articles, trade journal articles, and datasets). Students will be able to identify the strengths and weaknesses of these different source types. Students will be able to articulate how they would (or would not) make use of the information from these sources in real-world contexts (i.e., when working with future clients).

Assessment: The librarian/instructor can walk around the room and listen in on the groups' discussions to assess the students' engagement with and understanding of the activity. At the end of the session, the librarian/instructor leads the class in a discussion of the activity and addresses any questions the students may have. He/she can also collect the groups' worksheets and read through their responses after the session to determine whether the learning outcomes were met.

Activity: The librarian/instructor divides the class into groups of two or three students and explains the activity. Each group receives a worksheet with a real-world social work topic or problem/scenario. For example, a group might be told that they are a social worker at a hospital charged with selecting an effective intervention for new mothers experiencing postpartum depression.

Each group also receives three citations that will lead them to three different sources of information on their problem/scenario (if the session takes place in a classroom without computers, groups can be given printouts):

1. An article from a peer-reviewed social work journal
2. An article from a trade journal
3. A website, dataset, report, or policy document

Beginning with the first source, the groups are given 10 minutes to review each source and consider a set of questions. The librarian/instructor can give these questions to the students in the form of a worksheet or write them on a board or display them via a PowerPoint slide. Each group can designate one member as the group's recorder, who will either fill in the worksheet or take notes on paper or digitally. The questions/prompts are:

1. What type of source is this?
2. Briefly summarize the information provided by this source. Does it make use of or reference a particular methodology, theory, or practice model?
3. What do you perceive to be the source's strengths?
4. What do you perceive to be the source's weaknesses?
5. Can you use the information provided in this source to help your client(s)? Why or why not?

The librarian/instructor watches the time and walks around the room, listening in on the students' discussions. After the groups have worked through each of the three sources, the librarian/instructor leads the class in a discussion of the activity, and the groups can compare one another's experiences.

Evidence-Based Dentistry: Library Research

Contributors: Dorothy Ogdon, MSIS, AHIP (Assistant Professor, Reference, and Librarian & Liaison to the School of Dentistry, University of Alabama at Birmingham); and Carly T. McKenzie, PhD (Assistant Professor,

Department of Clinical and Community Sciences, University of Alabama at Birmingham, School of Dentistry)

Frame—Information Creation as a Process: This purpose of this lesson is to use information retrieval as the basis for critical reflection on the processes for gathering, creating, disseminating, and accessing scientific and health-related information. Other associated frames: Research as Inquiry and Searching as Strategic Exploration.

Target Audience: Students in the first year of the doctor of dental medicine degree. The lesson may be adapted for any graduate-level health sciences courses in evidence-based practice that include group research projects.

Setting: To be used in conjunction with a group research project that culminates in a team-based live debate. Students are assigned a debate topic and must conduct information-seeking activities to use in the live debate session. The team's performance in the debate is assessed by the course instructors.

Learning Outcomes: Students will develop an understanding of how information is created and disseminated by creating and implementing search strategies for PubMed and a resource of their choice. Students will select and reflect on the information creation process for two items discovered during their searching activities.

Assessment: Students will complete and submit a four-part group assignment designed to provide a framework for their searching activities. One complete form will be submitted by each group. The forms are used as a summative assessment following the librarian's in-class lectures and consultations with student groups.

Evidence-Based Dentistry Activity: Library Research

The activity is designed to be completed as a group assignment during designated class time or during group activities that take place outside of designated class time. The assignment should be completed as groups are conducting research for team-based writing or debate projects. A consultation session with a librarian is included as part of this assignment.

Working in your assigned debate team group, complete parts 1 and 2 of this form before the group consultation with the librarian. You may copy/paste search terms and other information from databases into this form. When copying/pasting a search, do not be concerned about text formatting; include enough information about your searching to facilitate informed discussion with the librarian. The group will submit a copy of this form with parts 1–4 completed after consultations with the librarian are finished.

Part 1. Identifying Search Terms: Copy and paste the complete text of your group debate topic. Working as a group, break the research question into component terms and complete the table below. Do not include terms that are not found in MeSH in the "Controlled Vocabulary" portion of the table. This portion of the table will be evaluated for accuracy. See table 3.3.

Part 2. Developing a PubMed Search: Begin exploring how your group will combine terms generated in part 1 to find the types of information described in the group responses to part 2. Draft a PubMed search strategy using combinations of terms from the table. Groups are encouraged to consider using additional tools or searching techniques such as filters, alternate MeSH terms, phrase searching, or wildcards when creating this search. Once you have drafted the search, respond to the prompts below.

1. Copy and paste the search string or search history here. Do not worry about formatting.
2. Did the search work well, or will it need revision? Write a three–five-sentence response that includes ideas from the group about what to change in the search to obtain more relevant results or questions about how to search for specific types of information or publications.

Table 3.3. Evidence-Based Dentistry: In-Class Group Activity

Main components and examples of clinical questions, according to their natures					
PICO(T) Component Patient, Population, Problem	Intervention (Exposure or Diagnostic Test)		Comparison (or Reference Standard)	Outcomes	Time
Search Strategy Development					
	Population	Intervention	Comparison	Outcomes	Time
Synonyms for terms/ potential search terms					
Terms from Controlled Vocabulary (MeSH)					

Part 3. Selecting Other Resources: Complete this part of the assignment before or after your consultation with the librarian. Select a second database or resource to use to locate information related to your assigned debate topic. You may select any resource your group feels is appropriate for your research topic except for PubMed Central or European PubMed Central. Consider selecting a resource that will provide results or information that may not be included in PubMed.

1. What resource did the group select? Provide the full name.
2. Explain why your group selected this resource to search in addition to PubMed. What types of information do you want to find using this resource? Is that information included in PubMed? Answer *yes* or *no* and support your answer with a three–five-sentence explanation.
3. Copy and paste the search strategy for the resource you selected. If you did not use a database, provide a one-sentence explanation of how you looked for information within the resource.
4. Review the information you found in the second resource and provide a response to both prompts:

    a. Are these results more or less useful for the group debate assignment than the results from PubMed? Explain why or why not.
    b. Are results from the PubMed search duplicated in the results from the second resource?

Part 4. Discussion of Results: Working in your assigned group, reflect on the searching activities for the group debate project. Select two items the group found while searching to use to respond to the prompts in this section.

1. Copy and paste or type the citation for an item from your PubMed search results here:
2. Respond to the following three questions:

    a. What type of information object is this item? Types of information objects include, but are not limited to, books, book chapters, journal articles, reports, websites, magazines, infographics, and personal communications.
    b. Give a general description of how the information provided in this information product was collected, reviewed, and made available to access.
    c. Why do you think information about this item was included in PubMed?

3. Select an item the group found using the second resource. Copy and paste or type the citation for the item here:
4. What was the name of the second resource your group searched for information?
5. Respond to the following three questions:

    a. What type of information object is this item? Types of information objects include, but are not limited to, books, book chapters, journal articles, reports, websites, magazines, infographics, and personal communications.
    b. Give a general description of how the information provided in this information product was collected, reviewed, and made available to access.
    c. Why do you think information about this item was included in the second resource the group used to find information?

As a group, discuss your experiences and observations about both the positive and negative aspects of the current systems for creating, disseminating, finding, and accessing scientific and health-related information. In the group's opinion, what could be improved? In the resources that are currently available what works well? Provide a three–five-sentence summary of the group discussion that includes specific examples from your searching activities.

Preparing for Publication

Contributor: Kelly A. Johnson, MS, DVM, MLIS (Veterinary Outreach and Information Resources Librarian, Flower-Sprecher Veterinary Library, Cornell University)

Frame—Information Creation as a Process: Students are asked to explore and evaluate opportunities for publication and for maximizing their scholarly impact.

Target Audience: Incoming veterinary residents. The lesson may also be adapted to other health sciences disciplines for which publication is an expected component of educational or professional programs.

Setting: To be used with incoming veterinary residents in preparation for publication. Residents are challenged to understand how to evaluate and execute the stages of the research cycle leading to impactful publication.

Learning Outcomes: Students will develop necessary investigative and critical skills to locate publishing and funding opportunities, select publishers, understand manuscript preparation, and maximize their visibility as research scientists.

Assessment: Students are asked to summarize their findings after each section by providing an example of the following, as is relevant to their research project:

- appropriate funding sources
- subject-appropriate journals
- a subject-appropriate journal that has been evaluated against criteria associated with predatory publishing (whether the student ultimately considers it predatory or not)
- manuscript parameters specific to their paper (citation style, word count, etc.)
- ORCiD ID

Activity: These exercises are designed to be completed individually in the classroom, with discussion following completion of each section. They could also be completed outside of the classroom prior to a discussion session.

Complete the following exercises using a topic you are currently researching, or, if you aren't currently working on a project, select a topic of interest.

Secure funding:

1. Grants.gov searches across multiple governmental funding agencies. Find a grant that fits within the scope of your research. Are you eligible for this grant?
2. Some organizations and foundations offer funding as well. Visit the websites of two or three professional organizations relevant to your area of research. Do any of them offer funding? Are you eligible for these grants?

Decide where to publish:

1. Visit the web pages of two or three journals, conferences, or professional organizations that are particularly relevant to your research. Are there calls for article submissions?
2. Search your topic in an academic database and note where similar research is being published. Are there journals that are particularly prevalent? (Many database filters allow you to view a ranked list of the journals that appear in your search.)
3. Using the name of an exemplary researcher, find where they are publishing (using their ORCiD identifier, web pages, or anywhere their publications are listed). Are they publishing heavily in any specific journals?

4. After selecting a journal you'd like to consider, find its aim and scope. Many journals make this information explicitly available somewhere on their web page. Is your research a good fit?
5. Find the journal's terms of publication. Who maintains copyright of your article? Is there a fee to publish? Are these terms acceptable to you?
6. If you are trying to publish something other than an original research article (e.g., case report, review article), does the journal accept that format?

Avoid predatory publishers. (For introductory information on predatory publishing, search PubMed for PMID 25657363. For this exercise, compare results from the journal you selected above against the *Journal of American Academic Research*; if this journal no longer exists, execute a web search to find another that has been identified as "predatory.")

1. Does the journal (or publisher) have a website? Does it look professional? Does it provide explicit information about the submission and editorial process?
2. Does the journal charge for publication? At what point is the author charged (at the time of submission or at the time of publication)?
3. Search two or more academic databases for the journal title. Do you get any results? Are they the kinds of results you would expect from an academic journal?
4. If the journal claims to be open access, is it included in the DOAJ (Database of Open Access Journals)?
5. Perform an internet search for the journal title (or publisher). What kinds of things do you see? Is there anything that makes you question the journal's validity?

Prepare your manuscript. Continue using the journal you selected above. On the journal's website, find author guidelines for submission.

1. Does the journal require a specific citation style?
2. Are there margin, font, or spacing requirements?
3. Is there a required format for tables and figures?
4. Are there file size restrictions for images?
5. Are you asked to remove authors' identifying information to allow for blind peer review?
6. Is there a word count limit for the manuscript? For the abstract?
7. Is the author asked to include a cover letter?

Make your research visible. ORCiD (orcid.org) identifiers are unique individualized codes assigned to researchers in order to link them to all their professional activities.

1. Using the name of a scholar in your field, find their ORCiD identifier by searching the ORCiD website (or you may find it anywhere they provide professional information, such as a website, a published paper, or LinkedIn).
2. Glance through the list of works displayed on their page. Do you see anything listed other than journal articles? Are there things that show up here that aren't likely to show up when you search their name in an academic database?
3. Is there an "Also known as" list provided on the page? Why is it beneficial for authors to include variants of their name, even if they have never changed it?
4. Register for your own ORCiD identifier (ORCiD is a free resource). Even if you don't have publications or other academic output to link to your account, you can populate the education and employment sections of your page. (If you prefer to keep your account private, you can restrict the visibility of your profile under Account Settings.)
5. Add a link to your ORCiD record anywhere that will maximize your academic visibility (on your LinkedIn profile, in your e-mail signature, etc.).

Chapter Four

Information Has Value

Librarians and researchers in the health sciences disciplines tend to understand the high cost of information in this field. Cost can mean price: individual journals can cost tens of thousands of dollars annually, and point-of-care tools that integrate into electronic health records (EHRs) and other hospital systems can reach seven figures quickly. Cost can also mean sacrifice: when libraries face a fiscal year promising a flat or decreased continuing resource budget, collection development teams must decide which resources can and must be sacrificed based on factors such as overall usage, cost per access, and the importance of the title in its discipline.

While cost is certainly associated with value, value is more of an inherent quality that goes beyond the monetary costs negotiated by those operating in the information marketplace. Value speaks to worth and importance, which can be subjective, but which definitely also have objective measures. Some of the defining attributes for information value in the health sciences include

- Publisher + Journal
- Information Platform: Print, Electronic, and Other
- Payment Model: Subscription or Open Access
- Accessibility: Library, Repository, and ILL
- Intellectual Property: Copyright, Citations, and Plagiarism
- Special Considerations: Predatory Publishing, Illegal Posting Sites, Third-World Voices, and Information Access in the Impoverished World

PUBLISHER + JOURNAL

Every discipline has top-tier journals and publishers. Discipline veterans will be familiar with these, as they have read and published in these journals and possibly even served on editorial boards. True to this chapter's frame, the articles published in these journals hold a very high value within the scholarly discourse. One could muse that the best way to determine a publisher's value is how much they charge for their journals; but the truth remains there are no definitive metrics in place to measure publisher impact. However, there are metrics to measure both journal and author impact within their discipline's scholarly discourse. Journal impact is measured by the impact that individual articles have upon the scholarly community. This is chiefly determined through the number of articles that are cited going forward, as well as the number of times those articles are cited. There are various models to determine the impact of a given journal, and resources that libraries and institutional research offices can subscribe to determine the same. These tools can allow researchers to quickly assess target journals for their manuscripts.

Having an idea of where an article will be submitted is important, as each journal will have specifications for submission that the author must observe while preparing the manuscript. Tools that rank journals allow authors to determine their first pick for submission, as well as any secondary journals if they face rejection with the first. As these resources base journal impact upon individual article impact, they can also be used to gauge the impact of specific authors within a discipline. This can be useful for department heads when determining the faculty members who are producing the most beneficial work within a given field or within their department. In addition to subscription resources, there are open access resources that can accomplish much the same purpose.

INFORMATION PLATFORM: PRINT, ELECTRONIC, AND OTHER

Accessibility of information can factor into its value. In today's global scholarship environment, health sciences researchers very often turn to electronic media first. When print was the primary platform for information delivery, supportive resources such as print indexes to periodical literature, annual review journals that summarized recent findings in a given discipline, and subject bibliographies were vital to library collections. The last 20 years of serials publishing has seen print journals with free online access turn into a primarily online publishing format. Print, if available, can come at additional cost, as can interactive modules and continuing education opportunities available on some publisher platforms.

PAYMENT MODEL: SUBSCRIPTION OR OPEN ACCESS

Two primary models exist for accessing information: subscriptions and open access. Subscription journal and book models often depend on the type and size of institutions and the number of potential users accessing any part of the subscription. Information is licensed, usually by a library, and use exists in the confines of a legally binding contract and usage agreement. Access to information is restricted by the subscription model, and access depends on one's affiliation with an institution and the amount of money the institution is willing to spend on the information resources. This "pay to play" model is not always fair or feasible, and it can severely restrict academic discourse since information is not always free, or even affordable. The open access model operates by asking authors to pay to have their research published, thereby making the information freely accessible by the academic community. Some disagreement exists among academics and librarians with some questioning the rigor of open access journal articles, while still others celebrate the opportunity open access presents for open information and open science.

ACCESSIBILITY: LIBRARY, REPOSITORY, AND ILL

Libraries are traditionally seen as the source for information across most disciplines. In addition to subscription packages to refereed journals and books, many libraries also maintain an institutional repository of publications by members of their parent institution. This makes scholarly research such as poster and paper presentations, dissertations and theses, and other types of scholarly activity available even without publishing in a journal. Most libraries also provide an invaluable service to the academic community by "loaning" owned materials from institution to institution in the form of interlibrary loan. If a library is part of a loaning community, lack of immediate access to a piece of information is solved by finding the item elsewhere.

INTELLECTUAL PROPERTY: COPYRIGHT, CITATIONS, AND PLAGIARISM

Placing value on information naturally relates to the intellectual integrity associated with copyright, proper use of citations, and plagiarism. While plagiarism can often be unintentional, it remains unethical and unprofessional. Violations of copyright and using copyrighted material without adequate citation not only devalues information but also tarnishes the life cycle of information sharing and the flow of ideas.

SPECIAL CONSIDERATIONS: PREDATORY PUBLISHING, ILLEGAL POSTING SITES, THIRD-WORLD VOICES, AND INFORMATION ACCESS IN THE IMPOVERISHED WORLD

Predatory publishing is not a new phenomenon but, rather, something that continues to plague the academic community. Coupled with ignorance of the problem and the desperation to publish, many academics have fallen prey to the clever tactics of predatory publishers. One method of determining an article's value is through its vetting by other scholars in that field via the peer-review process; this does not commonly happen when dealing with a predatory publisher.

While researchers' pressure to publish helps drive the predatory publishing business, illegal posting sites are driven by researchers' pressure to gain access to information that lies beyond their monetary ability to obtain. Illegal posting sites not only violate a journal and/or author's copyright but also can be used as a back door into unsuspecting users' computers and information networks. While the open access model has a noble purpose, illegal sites proliferate and undermine the good that can come from open access literature. Illegal posting sites have also become an unfortunate point of information access for some researchers and academics in third world, developing, and disadvantaged countries. Many people in these communities do not have the resources to acquire big-ticket subscription packages, and many struggle to perform research.

Third-world voices often have difficulty being heard in the scholarly discourse. The value of information is somewhat diminished when we look at the research that cannot be shared due to cost. Initiatives such as HINARI make strides toward equity of information access, but more work can be done in this area.

VALUE IN ACTION: CASE STUDIES

Contributing to the Conversation: The Value of Citations

Contributor: Alexandria Quesenberry, MSIS (Assistant Professor/Research & Learning Services Librarian, Health Sciences Library, University of Tennessee Health Science Center)

Frame—Information Has Value. Other associated frames: Scholarship as Conversation.

Target Audience: Undergraduate nursing (Accelerated BSN, BSN, RN-BSN). The lesson may also be adapted to other health sciences disciplines with an appropriate essay topic.

Setting: Undergraduate nursing students in the first writing-intensive course with an embedded librarian in an accelerated BSN program. Students

Value at a Glance: Quick Tips for Busy Librarians

Q: What is value?
A: The importance, worth, or usefulness of a type of information.

Information Has Value

Information possesses several dimensions of value, including as a commodity, as a means of education, as a means to influence, and as a means of negotiating and understanding the world. Legal and socioeconomic interests influence information production and dissemination.

http://www.ala.org/acrl/standards/ilframework

Types of Value:

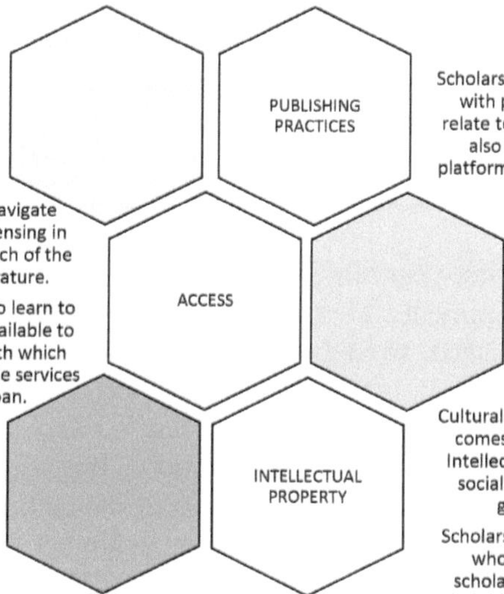

Scholars should familiarize themselves with publishers and journals that relate to their discipline. They should also learn to recognize reliable platforms of open access information.

Scholars must learn to navigate paywalls and resource licensing in order to gain access to much of the published scholarly literature.

It is to a scholar's benefit to learn to maximize the resources available to them through libraries with which they are affiliated, to include services such as interlibrary loan.

Cultural norms vary worldwide when it comes to copyright and plagiarism. Intellectual property falls under both social and legal standards within a given culture or country.

Scholars should be respectful of those who have gone before them in scholarly discourse, giving credit to their ideas and citing their words and ideas properly.

Special considerations for the health sciences:

- ❑ The NIH Public Access Policy, enacted in 2009, calls for open access publishing of NIH-funded peer-reviewed literature. [https://publicaccess.nih.gov/policy.htm] Consequently, scholars can find open access articles available within otherwise subscription-based journals.
- ❑ Scholars and authors in the health sciences should remain wary of predatory publishers when selecting journals for research or for publication. Librarians are on the forefront of helping scholars identify trustworthy information sources.

FRAMING HEALTHCARE 3

are familiar with searching library resources and databases from previous coursework. In this course, students are required to write an essay and cite their sources in the American Psychological Association (APA) style.

Learning Outcomes: After completion of this lesson, students will be able to:

- explain the importance of giving credit to the original authors/creators of ideas through proper citation,
- define plagiarism and how it is influenced by cultural and ethical values,
- participate in the community of scholarship through proper citation, and
- contribute to the scholarly conversation on horizontal violence through the creation of an essay.

Learning Activities

1. Citations and Plagiarism: What You Need to Know—a 15-minute lecture about the importance of giving credit to authors through citation, APA style, and plagiarism.
2. Exploring the Ethics of Plagiarism—a 5-minute to 10-minute group discussion about plagiarism, culture, and ethics. Students are provided with scenarios as part of a Think-Pair-Share learning strategy where they are paired up for discussion and share their thoughts with the class as part of a discussion. Example scenarios include the following:

    - Sally is a first-year nursing student and is having trouble with one of her assignments. Her friend David is in the same class and has already finished, so Sally asks to look over David's work and borrow ideas from it. Is this plagiarism?
    - You are peer-editing a fellow student's paper, and you notice that their paper doesn't have any citations, but you recognize phrases from your course textbook. As part of the editing process, you and the student have a discussion about each other's work. This student is international, and they explain to you that it isn't customary in their culture to reference the original author when using their words. How would you explain the importance of citing sources to your peer?

3. Contribute to the Conversation Using Citations:

    - This activity can be completed individually or as groups in class, or as a homework assignment outside of class time. After the lecture, students are given a scholarly article (Article A) about horizontal violence and asked to identify a piece of information cited in Article A. Students will then use the in-text citation to locate the full citation in Article A's reference list and locate the cited article (Article B) using the identifying information provided in the citation. Students are given the following worksheet:

After reading Article A, identify a sentence or two that the authors cited that you would like to use in your own essay on horizontal violence. Using the in-text citation, find the full citation in Article A's reference list and answer the following questions:

1. What sentence(s) did you find useful?
2. What is the number of the citation in the reference list?
3. As we discussed in class, not everything is cited in APA style. It is important for you to be able to identify the elements of a citation, even when it is not in APA style. Given that Article A is not written in APA style, identify the following information from the citation you selected in question 2:

    a. Author:
    b. Date:
    c. Article title:
    d. Journal title:
    e. Volume number:
    f. Page number(s):
    g. DOI/URL:

4. Using the information you identified above, locate the full text of the citation you selected.
5. Locate the information in the article that Article A cited and compare it to how it was reported in Article A. Is it an accurate scholarly conversation? Are there any differences or missing contexts?
6. Create APA-style citations for both articles to use in your essay assignment.

Assessment: Formative assessment can include the Think-Pair-Share discussion activity. Summative assessment includes the worksheet and eventual essay reference list.

When Databases Aren't Enough: The Paywall Problem

Contributors: Kimberly Tate-Malone, MLIS (Reference and Instruction Librarian, Seattle Central College); and Althea Lazzaro, MA, MLIS (Reference and Instruction Librarian, Seattle Central College)

Frame—Information Has Value. Other associated frames: Searching as Strategic Exploration.

Target Audience: Community college undergraduate allied health students (respiratory care, community health and education, health care services management). This lesson may also be adapted for other health sciences disciplines.

Setting: Lesson in an undergraduate credit-bearing information literacy course *or* one of a sequence of library workshops outside of a credit-bearing information literacy course.

Time: This lesson is designed for 2 instructional hours; it may also be adapted for online reading, lecture, and discussion.

Learning Outcomes

- Recognize systemic, personal, and community barriers to accessing needed information.
- Identify traditional and nontraditional search tools appropriate to information needs.
- Articulate the risks and rights associated with copyright, paywalls, and extralegal access to information.

Introduction

When we are teaching our third-year community college allied health students to use health sciences databases, it is with the knowledge that many of the settings in which they will (or already) work will not have access to the best evidence available due to the high cost of health sciences journals and databases. This comes into conflict with our emphasis on evidence-based medicine and the responsibilities that our students have toward the communities with which they work. The lack of access to needed evidence could have a detrimental impact on the well-being of patients and/or communities, and we want to equip our students to think critically about these potential consequences.

This lesson explores the economic realities of the health sciences information environment and how some researchers choose to go outside of traditional means of accessing information to ensure they are locating the best evidence for their practice. We do this by exploring the Sci-Hub/Libgen controversy (see “Materials”) and other ethical debates about access to information. We end by discussing the practicalities of extralegal access and its potential risks.

Students come away from this lesson with a deeper understanding of the barriers they face while searching, an awareness of the dissemination of knowledge in the health sciences, and new choices about how they will access information in the future.

Materials

- Copies of the Association of American Publishers' "Statement on Libgen/ Sci-Hub Complaint" and Aaron Swartz's "Guerilla Open Access Manifesto" *or* other pro/con sources for considering the ethics of traditional scholarly journal publishing and dissemination processes
- A computer with internet access
- Whiteboard and markers

Preparation

Students should have had a lesson on basic search skills and have searched for information on their topic using subscription databases and the free web. During this process, students should have noted when they couldn't gain access to a full text. This lesson works especially well when students are doing known item searching from a bibliography.

Session Instructions

1. Brief discussion of students' experiences of scholarly journal article and known item searching; prompt for feedback on barriers if not mentioned by students during discussion.

    a. Ask students why they were unable to access articles through search engines and/or library databases. Typical responses include hitting a paywall, author compensation, broken interface, user error, and inadequate library resources.

2. Short lecture on scholarly authorship and (non)compensation, traditional and alternative journal publishing (including open and gold access). *Peter Suber's* Open Access *is a great resource for understanding these concepts and is free from MIT Press. SPARC's (Scholarly Publishing and Academic Resources Coalition) website is good for more current material.*
3. Discussion of pros and cons of the traditional publishing model and extralegal access.

    a. Class reading (we use the popcorn method where students alternate reading aloud) of Aaron Swartz's "Guerilla Open Access Manifesto" and the Association of American Publishers' 2015 "Statement on Libgen/Sci-Hub Complaint."
    b. Check for comprehension of articles, explaining unknown terms, programs, etc.

c. Discuss questions raised by the readings *(choose a few from the following list)*: (1) How has access or a lack of access to information affected your ability to do your work as a professional? As a student? (2) What might having or not having access mean for the communities you are a part of or will be serving? (3) Is it ethical to access information extralegally? (4) Is it ethical for information to be limited to only those who can afford it? (5) Who do you think the authors of scholarly health sciences journal articles hope to reach? Do you think they are successful in their aim through the traditional journal publishing process? (6) What are some potential consequences of accessing articles extralegally? For example, redactions or updated drug dosage information can be missing from nonauthorized sources; ISP copyright letter; notice of service cancellation; or fines.

4. Brainstorm and demo alternative ways that scholars find and share scholarly work. For example, Sci-Hub, Library Genesis, ResearchGate, #icanhazpdf (on Twitter), reddit.com/r/scholar/, Google Scholar, author websites, institutional repositories, visiting other institutions, and e-mailing authors.
5. Describe practical considerations for accessing articles extralegally. For example, not using your home connection without a VPN or TOR client, using the public library (mention library resistance to disclosing user data), not logging in to personal accounts during search session, and such.
6. *Reflections/Assessment:* As a written reflection or in-class final discussion, pose these questions to students:

   a. When you're searching for evidence and come up against a paywall, what will you consider when deciding how to proceed with your research?
   b. After experiencing barriers such as paywalls as a researcher, would you make open access a priority when deciding how to publish your article as an author? Why or why not?

Lessons from the Lesson

We have found this lesson to be one of the most interesting class sessions that we teach. It's a moment when students recognize the structural and economic barriers that they have encountered in their research and that they will likely encounter as they continue in their profession. Once students can name those barriers, they engage in very interesting conversations about their personal ethics and the lengths to which they are willing to go to access the information they will need for their personal and professional practice.

Sweetening the Evidence

Contributor: Heather Brodie Perry, MLS (Reference Librarian/Assistant Professor, Stonehill College)

Frame—Information Has Value. Students are challenged to understand that funding source can influence the objectivity and credibility of research and to understand that the value of information as an economic driver should not be underestimated.

Target Audience: Graduate students in nutrition. The lesson may also be adapted for nursing students or any practitioners who may discuss popular reports of research with patients.

Setting: To be used in instructing graduate students in evaluating research in preparation for performing research or working with patients.

Learning Outcomes: Students will better understand how information resources reflect their creators' expertise and credibility, and they will understand that information must be critically evaluated. Students will learn that information has several dimensions of value including as a tool for marketing or thwarting regulations.

Activity: In the 1950s, concerns emerged about the potential links between sugar and heart disease; these concerns threatened sugar's market share. To address these concerns, the Sugar Research Foundation recruited and paid Harvard researchers to publish a 1967 review of studies cherry-picked to minimize the role of sugar and implicate dietary fat in the development of coronary heart disease (O'Connor, 2016). This research proved problematic in obscuring the truth about the role of sugar in the development of cardiovascular disease (CVD), denying consumers the opportunity to make informed decisions about dietary choices. The industry continued to support research exonerating sugars, and by the 1980s, the dietary guidelines focused on the reduction of dietary fats to address concerns about heart disease. Many of the emerging low-fat products replaced fat with sugars. Decades later, the American Heart Association now recognizes the role of excess sugar consumption in the worldwide epidemics of obesity and CVD (Johnson et al., 2009), and recommends limiting consumption of added sugars.

Industry influence on research is not limited to research into sugars but extends across many issues in nutrition and health. Industry-sponsored research is associated with pro-industry conclusions (Bekelman, Li, & Gross, 2003), but bias is not always recognized. The research finds that study outcomes can be correlated with funding source; however, conflict of interest disclosure statements may not provide readers with the information they need to evaluate the quality of the research. Readers should focus on the scientific merit of the research including the methods, data, results, and conclusions, while also considering how financial relationships can affect research in negative, neutral, and positive ways (Resnik & Elliott, 2013). Readers are required to make informed decisions about the quality of the research and the potential for bias from funding source, rather than simply rejecting all funded research.

Media reports on recent health studies frequently report benefits without explaining the limitations of a study. Research in the lab may not translate into real-life conditions. Industry may see impacts that are more positive on their bottom line than on public health. Health studies should be approached with a critical stance to avoid being taken in by information that is too good to be true.

1. Find a popular media report of a recent study; for example, Google the terms *red wine* and *study*. Examine the popular report.

    - What claims are being made?
    - Are the strengths and limitations of the study described?
    - Is the funding source of the study stated?

2. Use clues in the article to trace the study referred to in the popular report back to the original study.

    - Was the methodology appropriate to the research questions? Are the studies observational studies or double-blind clinical trials?
    - Are the conclusions well supported by the findings?

3. Does the media report accurately report the study?
4. Search a disciplinary database such as PubMed, CINAHL, Web of Science, or Google Scholar for the topic of the study (i.e., wine).

    - What is the scientific consensus on the topic?
    - Did you examine the articles for funding disclosure?
    - Does the media report present a narrative that is more exciting than the current scientific consensus on the issue?

Assessment: At the conclusion of the session, have students complete a one-minute paper answering the questions: What will you consider when determining the credibility of an information resource? How has your understanding of evaluating information expanded through this exercise?

References

Bekelman, J. E., Li, Y., & Gross, C. P. (2003). Scope and impact of financial conflicts of interest in biomedical research: A systematic review. *Journal of the American Medical Association, 289*(4), 454–465.

Johnson, R. K., Appel, L. J., Brands, M., Howard, B. V., Lefevre, M., Lustig, R. H., Sacks, F., Steffen, L. M., & Wylie-Rosett, J. (2009). Dietary sugars intake and cardiovascular health: A scientific statement from the American Heart Association. *Circulation, 120*(11), 1011–1020.

O'Connor, A. (2016, September 13). Sugar backers paid to shift blame to fat. *The New York Times*, p. A1.

Resnik, D. B., & Elliott, K. C. (2013). Taking financial relationships into account when assessing research. *Accountability in Research, 20*(3), 184–205.

Communicating with APA: Writing and Citing for Graduate Nursing Students

Contributor: Katelyn Quirin Manwiller, MLIS (Public Services and Assessment Librarian, Trexler Library, DeSales University)

Frame—Information Has Value. Students will be prompted to discuss in small groups the value of using research in written assignments and the importance of citation. They are given an overview of the APA style guide and asked to address a series of formatting and citation prompts. Other associated frames: Scholarship as Conversation.

Target Audience: Part-time, graduate nursing (MSN, DNP). The lesson may also be adapted to undergraduate nursing or other health sciences disciplines using appropriate citation styles.

Setting: To be used with part-time graduate nursing students in preparation for formal writing assignments, including dissertations. Students are required to adhere to the APA style guide. The lesson can be used virtually or in the classroom.

Learning Outcomes: Students will recognize the value of information and its communication in their professional and academic work. Students will be able to correctly format and cite using the APA style guide.

Assessment: Formative assessment for this lesson includes responses to in-class discussion, group verbal response to the activity, and/or individual response to the activity via a worksheet. Summative assessment for this lesson could be librarian review of reference lists submitted for assignment.

Activity: Information and APA

This activity can be completed in class individually, in groups, or as a large class discussion prompted by the librarian.

Part 1. Understanding the Value of Information.

Discussion questions:

- What information is valued in the daily work of a nurse?
- Why is it important?
- How do you communicate it?
- What information is valued in your academic work?
- How does it compare to the information in your professional work?

Read the following passage from *Standards for Privacy of Individually Identifiable Health Information; Final Rule*:

> Congress recognized the importance of protecting the privacy of health information given the rapid evolution of health information systems in the Health Insurance Portability and Accountability Act of 1996 (HIPAA), Public Law 104-191, which became law on August 21, 1996. HIPAA's Administrative Simplification provisions, sections 261 through 264 of the statute, were designed to improve the efficiency and effectiveness of the health care system by facilitating the electronic exchange of information with respect to certain financial and administrative transactions carried out by health plans, health care clearinghouses, and health care providers who transmit information electronically in connection with such transactions. To implement these provisions, the statute directed HHS to adopt a suite of uniform, national standards for transactions, unique health identifiers, code sets for the data elements of the transactions, security of health information, and electronic signature.

Decide if the following examples are cited correctly:

- The Administrative Simplification provisions of HIPAA were designed to make the electronic exchange of health care information more efficient.
- The Department of Health and Human Services adopted "uniform, national standards" for the transmission of medical records (Health Insurance Portability and Accountability Act of 1996, 2002).
- Under federal law, Americans have a right to certain privacy protections.

Part 2. Communicating Your Information.

Discussion questions:

- Are there regulations in how you communicate information in your job? If so, why do you think those regulations exist?
- Why is it important to follow regulations in academic communication?
- What is the value of using the APA style guide for the writing and formatting of your work?

Writing Style: Rewrite these sentences in active voice:

- The final exam was failed by one-third of the class.

- The participants were asked to fill out a survey by the researcher.
- The patient records should have been reviewed by the nurse.

Page Formatting: Correctly implement APA style for the following examples:

- *Title Page:* Using the example title of "Information Has Value: The Importance of APA," format a title page.
- *Headings:* Format the headings of a "Method" section with one Level 1 heading, two Level 2 headings, and two Level 3 headings.
- *Citations:* Correct the mistakes in these reference list citations:

Lockwood, C. What is the Best Nursing Handover Style to Ensure Continuity of Information for Hospital Patients? (2016). *International Journal of Nursing Studies, 58*, pp. 97-99.

Martin, Colin and David Thompson. 2000. *Design and analysis of clinical nursing research studies.* London: Routledge.

Summary of the HIPAA Privacy Rule. (2003). U.S. Department of Health & Human Services. Retrieved on September 16, 2018 from https://www.hhs.gov/sites/default/files/privacysummary.pdf

Gagnon, K. & Sabus, C. (2015). Professionalism in a digital age: Opportunities and considerations for using social media in health care. Physical Therapy, *95*(3), 406-414. DOI:10.2522/ptj.20130227

Evidence-Based Practice: Pathways to the Information

Contributor: Ann Hallyburton, MSLS, MPH, AHIP, CHIS (Research and Instruction Librarian / Liaison to the Health and Human Sciences, Hunter Library, Western Carolina University)

Frame—Information Has Value

Target Audience: Postgraduates and professionals across health care disciplines.

Setting: Instruction may take place online asynchronously or synchronously or in a physical classroom. Course incorporates readings, videos, and exercises.

Learning Outcomes: Individuals who take the course should be able to:

1. provide a basic definition of evidence-based practice information;
2. differentiate between research study designs forming the basis for evidence-based practice (EBP) publications;
3. construct effective searches using parts of a clinical PICO (Patient, Population, or Problem; Intervention; Comparative intervention; desired or dreaded Outcome) question;
4. choose tools and methods appropriate for locating relevant information; and
5. understand the necessity of questioning information sources, even those from eminent organizations, researchers, or journals.

Assessment: If conducted solely online, short quizzes may be embedded throughout. If assessment and/or quiz functionality is not readily available, instructors may employ features available within resources commonly used within libraries (e.g., Poll function within SpringShare's *LibGuides*, free resources within SurveyMonkey, etc.).

If conducted in person, instructors may use a game-based learning platform (e.g., Kahoot!). Initial assessment focuses on participants' grasp of EBP and understanding of relevant study and publication types. Instructors may choose to cover introductory materials in less detail if most participants grasp foundational concepts. Short question-answer segments are interspersed throughout.

Activity: PICO—P, PI, PO Search

Sections within activity should be completed sequentially. If asynchronous and self-paced, learners may choose to leave off the latter parts of the activity depending upon need. If conducted synchronously, instructors may also choose to omit parts depending upon the needs of target populations.

Overview of EBP Information Types

- Provide a brief overview of EBP. Direct participants to view 4-minute video "Evidence-informed practice" from the Ontario Centre of Excellence (https://youtu.be/Xiv75BLGtrs).
- Review most common publication types emanating from EBP research: systematic reviews, meta-analyses, and research articles providing the findings of randomized controlled trials, cohort and other retrospective studies, and case studies. Duke University Medical Center's Library and Archives provides a good overview (https://guides.mclibrary.duke.edu/ebptutorial).
- View 2-minute video "Systematic Review and Meta-analysis" from the University of Maine System's University College Off-Campus Library Services (https://youtu.be/04E8JiXY2s4).

Example assessment question: What research type requires researchers to systematically appraise as much relevant research as they (and their information professionals) can find to determine what most of the well-conducted research suggests?

- Randomized controlled trial
- **Systematic review**
- Narrative review

PICO

- Watch 3-minute video “2 X 4 Word Searching with the PICO Clinical Question” (https://youtu.be/s1OmlKJ4Ws0) from Western Carolina University’s Ann Hallyburton.
- Download “P–PO” worksheet to aid in mapping initial search terms and alternate search terms discovered through search process (https://researchguides.wcu.edu/ld.php?content_id=42875095).
- Review clinical question components. If conducting class synchronously, prompt participants to provide example questions. Draw from examples to pinpoint words to be used in searching.

Example assessment question: What are the parts of the PICO clinical question?

- Patient; Impatient; Calm; Overzealous
- Pizza; Ice cream; Chocolate; Oreos
- **Patient, population, problem; Intervention; Comparative intervention; Outcome**

Searching with P, PI, and PO

Systematic review searching tools: Take terms identified in PICO process and use within systematic review search tools such as Cochrane Library’s Cochrane Reviews (https://www.cochranelibrary.com/cdsr/reviews) and Campbell Collaboration Online Library (https://www.campbellcollaboration.org/library.html), both of which offer a great deal of free access.

Guideline searching tools: Review professional practice guideline resources for relevant practice areas. Such guidelines are often available through professional organizations, federal and state governments, and the World Health Organization. The Publication Type limiter within PubMed’s Advanced Search Builder also offers options for “guideline” and “practice guideline” searching. Cover resources relevant to target populations.

Instructors may also mention Guideline Central (https://www.guidelinecentral.com) tools and ECRI Institute’s Guidelines Trust (https://guidelines.ecri.org), resources attempting to fill the void left by the closure of the Agency for Healthcare Research and Quality’s National Guideline Clearinghouse (NGC). [For individuals unfamiliar with NGC, background is relevant as many resources still refer to NGC. NGC provided a freely accessible repository for clinical guidelines with the added value of stringent inclusion criteria, frequent updating, Food and Drug Administration drug warnings, and cross-guideline summaries. The resource ceased being updated in July 2018 due to funding cuts.]

Use tools that search across literature types like freely available PubMed and Google Scholar and subscription databases like CINAHL and EMBASE. Add words describing desired study type (e.g., "systematic," "randomized") to PICO components.

Questioning information: View 13-minute TED video "What Doctors Don't Know about the Drugs They Prescribe" by Ben Goldacre (https://www.ted.com/talks/ben_goldacre_what_doctors_don_t_know_about_the_drugs_they_prescribe?utm_campaign=tedspread&utm_medium=referral&utm_source=tedcomshare).

Example assessment question: Is it likely that someone can find *all* the research ever conducted on a health or human care issue?

Yes

No

Chapter Five

Research as Inquiry

Elizabeth Yost and Marianne Sade

"RESEARCH AS INQUIRY" IN THE ACADEMIC CONTEXT: BACKGROUND

The Research as Inquiry frame states: "Research is iterative and depends upon asking increasingly complex or new questions whose answers in turn develop additional questions or lines of inquiry in any field" (Framework, 2015). This frame encourages researchers to learn how to delve into topics. This skill is often built early in college through increasingly complex research assignments or semester-long research projects. Learning how to ask relevant questions and dig through years of research is key in successfully completing research assignments correctly and in a timely fashion. Asking preliminary questions is only one key part of this frame. Perhaps more important is the emphasis on asking new questions to see where scholars have not yet found answers and where new research can be completed. The ACRL Framework suggests eight knowledge practices and nine dispositions to help learners sharpen skills.

Health sciences is arguably one of the most dynamic research areas today. Educating students in the idea that "Research as Inquiry" is key for them to be able to constantly check and recheck; as new research is added, old assumptions of health change, and technology becomes more pervasive. New questions ought to be asked, and areas that are outdated ought to be challenged. To do so, though, requires a good command of the knowledge skills and dispositions listed within this framework. Being able to work with conflicting information, the first knowledge practice within the framework, is useful as science and technology change the field. Determining the scope of the investigation is useful as the knowledge will expand and the focus should be redrawn frequently. Breaking down questions is key in evaluating the overall idea of health or health care as these are far too large to be tackled within research questions. Each of the knowledge practices and dispositions within the Research as Inquiry framework is uniquely primed for health sciences research models. This chapter will discuss the implications of the frame as part of a broad and inclusive health sciences education as well as the experience of using elements of the Research as Inquiry frame as part of a larger grant experience with a first-year seminar within an interdisciplinary health sciences course.

One example of how a small-sized liberal arts college addressed this frame can be seen in a collaboration between a faculty librarian, referred to as librarian through this work, and a faculty member at Washington College in a first-year seminar, "Health and Technology." This collaboration was part of a larger grant experience with a group of five colleges who received an Institute of Museum and Library Services SPARKS Ignite grant, titled *Information Literacy Framework Cooperative Project for At-Risk Student Success in Smaller Colleges* (for more information, see https://digitalcommons.ursinus.edu/imls_ilframework/7/). The efforts were focused on the role of librarians using framework-focused instruction to improve outcomes for at-risk, first-year students. At Washington College, ACRL frames were used to help develop four learning outcomes that would lay a research foundation for the students during their health-based first-year seminar (FYS). Classroom activities focused on supporting skills and concepts that at-risk students might need to move up to a "starting line" or be on more equal footing with their peers. The instruction librarians concentrated on these four outcomes to shape pedagogy and lesson plans. Each institution was free to use or adapt these lessons as they saw fit given the variety in scale of participation.

The Partnership

Washington College is a small liberal arts college on the Eastern Shore of Maryland. Like many institutions of higher education, special courses are required of first-year students to help integrate them into the college curriculum. These first-year seminars (FYS) consist of no more than 18 students and are designed to teach critical inquiry, college-level writing, presentation, and research skills. The Research as Inquiry frame naturally aligns with skills that students are encouraged to master in these courses. Part of the requirements for these courses entails working with librarians to introduce students to research resources available at the college. These partnerships with the librarians are crucial not only to the success of the courses but also to the success of students throughout their college education. By creating an understanding of the library, the resources found there, and the role of librarian in the research process, students can build their information-literacy skills. Research supports this integration as a best practice for teaching information literacy skills (Beutter Manus, 2009). Though methods and format of research differ among disciplines, information literacy and research inquiry skills are necessary throughout all disciplines and are often significantly lacking in first-year students.

"Health and Technology" is an interdisciplinary course that explores the impact technology has on physical, mental, and social health by examining types of technology, technological history, and differences in adoption and use among demographic groups. The main research project in this course is a traditional, journal-style article that answers the question "Does technology impact health?" Students carry out independent research over 12 weeks that assesses health outcomes (physical, mental, and social) using three new applications (apps). The research paper showcases their own data as well as a comprehensive literature review of existing research on the impact of technology on health. Students have the opportunity to consider that there was no correct response or path to their research assignment but, rather, that searching for reliable information in the health field in particular can radically change. This encourages them to ask more questions more often. The course is well suited for the Research as Inquiry framework, as the topic is ever-changing and researchers are constantly evolving their understanding of the impact of apps on health outcomes. Students being able to evaluate competing claims within the research exposes them to additional opportunity to ask questions.

To best address the Research as Inquiry component, the faculty member and librarian worked together to design specific learning outcomes for the course, which included:

- understanding that research is an iterative, multistage process, and
- understanding and utilizing utilization of library services.

In addition to data gathered from pre- and post-tests of information literacy, qualitative data was also gathered to assess the impact of the librarian-embedded intervention. The librarian participated in both the classroom and online portions of the course and was assigned key components of the course that helped students explore the idea of "research as inquiry" and other information literacy skills. Students met with the librarian four times throughout the semester both as a group and in one-on-one sessions/consultations to build a rapport. Both the faculty member and librarian were able to identify gaps in student understanding of the research process early on through an exercise during the first library instruction where students described their research process. By the end of the class, students reviewed and identified areas where they could adjust their research strategies and more easily access and utilize library resources. Additionally, the "at-risk" students had the most significant improvement between pre- and post-test scores of information literacy.

Expectations and Outcomes

Although the framework is broad in scope, touching many academic levels, this work focused on the basics for first-year students: scaffolding for the future and getting them prepared for the academic discourse within and between disciplines. They first needed an appreciation for the practice of breaking complex broader considerations into smaller chunks or questions. Beginning to think in these terms is a challenge for first-year students.

The Research as Inquiry frame's objectives were crucial to helping students begin to understand the complexities of the iterative nature of research on an academic level. The following objectives were integrated into the course curriculum:

1. Objective 1: Learners will apply the information-seeking process.

    - Step 1: Understand the information-seeking process, that there are multiple steps, and that it is iterative.
    - Step 2: Determine where to seek information for a need and understand what each option might provide.
    - Step 3: Develop search strategies that support the information need.

2. Objective 2: Learners will recognize the librarian as a go-to person for research help.

    - Framework Disposition: Learners who are developing their information-literate abilities seek appropriate help when necessary.

"Learners will apply the information-seeking process. Step 1: Understand the information-seeking process, that there are multiple steps, and that it is iterative." The frame specifically outlines that there are "multiple steps" in the research process and that research is iterative in nature. When designing the learning-centered in-class library instruction for Washington College, engaging the students in a reflective activity as early as possible in the semester was key to understanding their base level understanding of what the research process involved.

The first activity was one in which students began by considering their "research process," and then they wrote, drew, outlined, or described their process. Students then identified any issues they encountered in their research process. The results were surprising in that most of their replies detailed their *writing* process with little attention to characterizing how they go about doing the research. Most of the iterative steps involved writing and draft revisions before turning in a final paper. It could be that they had never thought about their research process to this extent. Seeing where the students were coming from emphasized the importance of the Research as Inquiry frame for this course.

After a short discussion of student work and the overall idea of research as a process, the students watched *Picking Your Topic* Is *Research*, a short film with film guide that reinforced the iterative nature of research. (Multimedia referenced in this lesson are available via our IMLS Toolkit of Learning Activities: https://digitalcommons.ursinus.edu/imls_ilframework/.) After another brief discussion, they revisited their work and had the chance to change their depictions, noting how they could improve their research process using their newfound knowledge—thus reinforcing the iterative nature of the process.

In preparation for the second class together, students were assigned to watch *The Information Cycle* video that was reviewed during the face-to-face class time. After this, students participated in a quick exercise to introduce a research publication time line as a threshold concept. Several students were given science-related print sources when they entered class, and for the exercise, they were asked to line themselves up in order of publication from longest to produce/oldest (i.e., book) to shortest to produce/newest (i.e., a printed tweet). This was critical since their major class assignment focused on using the most current information on the impact of technology on health outcomes.

This class primarily addressed the importance of noting the sources for health sciences–based research and featured group projects that examined a variety of source types, including news, websites, tweets, and journal articles on the topic "Are Oreo cookies addictive?" Our discussion considered popular and scholarly outlets and supporting evidence (or lack of) for reliable information that they could apply to their own "app" research paper for the course.

Reinforcing the "iterative" nature of this frame was significant as it was observed firsthand that students were surprised that they would most likely need to revisit and refine their search strategies now that they were in a more rigorous academic environment. They were beginning to understand that higher-quality results would be expected from their search strategies and that they were unlikely to find these results using a simple Google search.

"Learners will apply the information-seeking process. Step 2: Determine where to seek information for a need and understand what each option might provide." To delve deeper into their search processes during their final face-to-face class with the librarian, the class was flipped, and the librarian asked students to watch a video on "Search Strategies and Methods" and answer prompts. In class, they completed a worksheet that started with a mind map

to help them develop search terms that would find relevant, peer-reviewed articles in the library's database. It became a path to defining their questions about their personal health application research papers. They named terms and then tried them out through searches. If they needed better results, they consulted their maps and tried other terms. In addition, they were asked to explore subject terms that were linked to search results in an attempt to broaden their keyword strategy. Students began to explore how this multidisciplinary search product works.

It is important that librarians establish themselves as approachable research experts who are willing to assist students during their critical first semester. Students were frequently reminded that librarians were their guides on how to best access the information they needed. Part of this was done through the one-on-one meetings, but it was also reiterated frequently in class and in meetings with the faculty member or through written feedback on paper drafts.

"Learners will apply the information-seeking process. Step 3: Develop search strategies that support the information need." To complete this objective, students were asked to reflect back on previous sessions. Basic mind mapping—concept mapping—as well as reflecting on/asking the "five *W*'s" (who, what, when, where, and why?) helped reinforce their own strategies. Students used the map to brainstorm and use words from it to begin a practice search. Students were reminded to consider the types of sources they saw and to reflect back on whether their source was suitable to their assignment. All questions librarian instructors ask as prompts help students develop and subsequently refine their search strategies.

Critical thinking is an important part of this process. Students need to be able to digest what they find, sort through search results, and reflect on the relevance of the information to their topic. Students need to be able to consider whether their original question needs to change based on what they discovered. Reading, not just skimming, is a major part of how students slowly digest information and become more expert on their topic of interest. As they master these skills, they can more clearly plan their strategy. Deep dives into the literature are daunting for most first-year students but are fundamental to a successful academic experience in the health sciences. At times, it was important to reassure them they were not getting lost along the way.

"Learners will recognize the librarian as a go-to person for research help." Classwork designed for this outcome was critical to pitch the librarian as students' research coach from day one. The course concentrated on getting students to see the librarian as their guide. Our inspiration was the Research as Inquiry's disposition: "Learners who are developing their information-literate abilities seek appropriate help when necessary" (Framework, 2015)

The course required them to meet with their librarian individually during the first week. During these meetings, students discussed their former experience with doing research (e.g., did they have a high school library/librarian experience?) and talked about their possible strategy to choose their research topic for the semester. Mostly it was an opportunity for the librarian to get to know the students and for students to get to know their librarian. These one-on-one, in-person meetings made it clear that students were more inclined to interact with the librarian outside of class. Observational assessment shows overall resistance of incoming students to ask for research assistance.

Lessons and Next Steps

Having a collaborative partnership between the faculty member and librarian where focused time and energy was directed onto the same group of students was paramount to the success of this work. Advance planning during the break before the semester was key for the faculty member and librarian to get to know each other, discuss pedagogy, create learner-centered activities both in class and online, construct grade rubrics, and fully integrate the objectives in the syllabus.

Thinking about the research process and observing firsthand that students did not have experience reflecting on their process was crucial knowledge to have at the start of the course where the major assignment was a research paper on a current health craze. Because of this, the professor and librarian were able to focus on helping students see the iterative process that good research requires. The iterative process of research was revisited from different points during the semester and reinforced through individual and class work assignments.

From the librarian's perspective, this was a rich opportunity to partner with faculty to create assignments, be embedded in the classroom, and see firsthand the complexity of students' approaches to research through numerous lenses. From the faculty perspective, the connecting of the students to the librarian and the formal relationship this project constructed was necessary for the students to be able to fully carry out independent research at the collegiate level. It also allowed the faculty member a better understanding of how to verbalize the ideas within the framework. Often, simplifying something that is an everyday action—such as research to a faculty member—can be difficult, and having a professional and a framework helped break down the process into manageable tasks for first-year students.

Time constraints and the nature of a busy fall semester were the biggest challenges in this experience. Additional time was needed to meet with each student individually to build trust and introduce the idea that librarians are there to help with each step of the research process. The librarian and faculty member learned that planning more time on the development of certain assignments, as well as introducing more assignments up front, might have been more helpful to the students.

There was an assumption that students were comfortable and competently skilled at doing high school–level research, such that minimal time would be needed for them to understand the difference between high school level and college level. However, their skills varied greatly, and even more remedial approaches or tutorials may have been useful to some of the class. More time spent on evaluating recent science and pseudoscience websites would have also benefited students. Because the topic of this class is relatively new and there is an abundance of research being published on the impact of apps on health outcomes with little agreement, this course was an excellent one to implement the Research as Inquiry frame.

RESEARCH AS INQUIRY IN FIRST-YEAR INTERDISCIPLINARY HEALTH SCIENCES COURSES

Overall, students showed immense gains in their information literacy skills from the partnership. The emphasis and additional attention devoted to helping first-year students better understand health research is paramount as we train the next generation of health care professionals. In order to address major health problems, health care professionals need to be able to conduct iterative research that helps them discover the diverse views that can be found in the research. For this course, having students learn that there was no "right answer" and that research generally poses more questions than it answers allowed students to see the nuanced ways that technology can impact their health: sometimes good, sometimes bad, and sometimes indistinguishable. Their health, like technology, is changing, and there are multiple factors to consider. In viewing the research process through this ACRL frame, the knowledge practices and dispositions posed by the faculty/librarian partnership will serve these students well in their continued educational pursuits.

REFERENCES

Beutter Manus, S. J. (2009). Librarian in the classroom: An embedded approach to music information literacy for first-year undergraduates. *Notes, 66*(2), 249–261. Music Library Association. Retrieved July 19, 2018, from Project MUSE database.

Framework for Information Literacy for Higher Education. American Library Association. February 9, 2015. https://www.ala.org/acrl/standards/i/framework, accessed August 22, 2018.

INQUIRY IN ACTION: CASE STUDIES

Research Matters: Asking the Question

Contributors: Heather Healy, MA, MLS (Clinical Education Librarian, Hardin Library for the Health Sciences, University of Iowa); and Kate Karacay (Senior Academic Advisor, University of Iowa)

Frame—Research as Inquiry. Other associated frames: Information Creation as Process. Students learn about formulating research questions and about types of information sources from two online modules from New Literacies Alliance (NLA) completed before class. At class, students are challenged to apply these concepts to new scenarios.

Target Audience: Undergraduate pre-health students, including pre-medicine, pre–physician assistant, and pre-dentistry. The lesson may be adapted to other health sciences disciplines.

Setting: Lesson for library instruction for first-semester students taking a first-year seminar class that explores the health care careers of doctors, physician assistants, and dentists.

Learning Outcomes: Students will create a list of characteristics to consider when identifying and choosing information sources. Students will analyze research scenarios to assess the appropriate scope of a research question.

Assessment: Quizzes in the NLA modules are scored and can be used as formative or summative assessment. Class discussion following group activities about focusing research questions and differentiating information types provides formative assessment. Completed worksheets and charts can be collected for summative assessment.

Activities

Flipped classroom exercise. Before attending the session, students complete the following two NLA modules: *Ask the Right Questions* and *Types of Information*. The framework-based lessons are offered under CC-BY-NC-SA licenses and are available at https://newliteraciesalliance.org.

Research question exercise. Building from the "Ask the Right Questions" lesson completed before class, students work in pairs to examine one of the research scenarios that follow. (The reference to "library search tool" in these scenarios can be replaced with an appropriate local resource, such as a discover layer or database.) Students assess the scope and effectiveness of the research question by completing a brief worksheet.

- *Research Scenario 1:* Valeria plans to investigate the importance of handwashing for physicians. She uses her library's search tool and retrieves more than 3,500 results. In skimming the first page of results, she sees many articles that look promising, but the results are on a wide variety of

Inquiry at a Glance: Quick Tips for Busy Librarians

Q: What is inquiry?
A: Focusing attention on an unresolved question in a given discipline or between two or more disciplines.

Research as Inquiry

Research is iterative and depends upon asking increasingly complex or new questions whose answers in turn develop additional questions or lines of inquiry in any field.

http://www.ala.org/acrl/standards/ilframework

Inquiry Process:

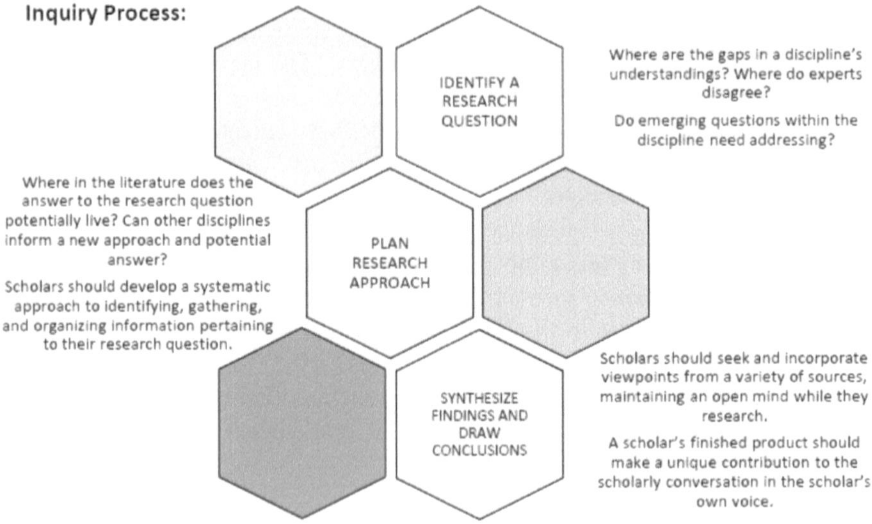

Special considerations for the health sciences:

- ❑ Health sciences professionals incorporating the expertise of colleagues from fellow health-related disciplines is a key component of interprofessional practice and patient-centered care.
- ❑ Many health sciences journals are highly selective, with very low acceptance rates. To increase chances of acceptance, scholars should ensure that they are addressing a question of import that is not sufficiently answered in recent literature when submitting an article for publication.

topics related to handwashing, such as compliance, concerns of patients, proper technique, and such.

- *Research Scenario 2:* Ethan plans to investigate the following research question: What effect can patients have on health care providers' compliance with handwashing guidelines? He uses the library's search tool and finds articles that discuss how patients may increase provider compliance,

others that relate to patient safety, and still others that examine patients' handwashing techniques.
- *Research Scenario 3:* Deirdre hopes to learn the most effective method for hand hygiene. After exploring the topic using the library's search tool, she finds articles detailing the effectiveness of alcohol-based hand rubs while other articles describe the importance of handwashing. She also finds discussions about which products assure better compliance.
- *Research Scenario 4:* Dinesh wants to answer this question: How does the wearing of artificial fingernails affect the hand hygiene of dentists? In looking over initial search results using the library's search tool, he retrieves many results related to contact dermatitis and other allergic reactions to artificial nails.

Worksheet

- Has this researcher used a well-developed research question?
- Why or why not?
- How might the researcher change the question?
- Based on your suggestions, rewrite the research question.

After the worksheets are complete, the whole class can discuss how the questions could be changed to adjust the scope of the inquiry. Additionally, the scenarios allow for discussions of how the researchers might proceed to narrow their search, deal with conflicting information, or deal with a lack of information.

Information types exercise. Building from the "Types of Information" lesson completed before class, students work in groups to develop a list of characteristics to differentiate source types. The instructor gives each group an article (print or online) from a popular, trade, or scholarly health sciences publication. For example, articles from *MedlinePlus Magazine*, *Dentistry Today*, and the *Journal of the Academy of Physician Assistants* would work well. (Other choices based on available resources and students' disciplines would also work.)

Each group records notes in a chart (a completed example follows; see table 5.1). After completion, the whole class discusses the characteristics identified by each group and how the observed qualities of those characteristics vary by source type. If students struggle with developing a list, the instructor can give them a partial or whole list of characteristics.

Reference: Treating rheumatoid arthritis: Search for a cure. (2018, July 18). *MedlinePlus Magazine*. Retrieved from https://magazine.medlineplus.gov/article/treating-rheumatoid-arthritis-search-for-a-cure

Library 101: Introduction to Health Sciences Resources

Contributors: Irma Quiñones (Associate Professor, Health Sciences Librarian, University of Memphis); and Brannen Vick Varner (Assistant Professor, Research and Instructional Services Librarian, University of Memphis)

Frame—Research as Inquiry. Students realize that research can be done in many ways, through many databases and library services. Other associated frames: Information Has Value.

Target Audience: Undergraduate nursing students. The lesson may also be adapted to any other health sciences disciplines that require research and information needs.

Setting: In-person, one-shot instruction to introduce health sciences resources to undergraduate first-year nursing students.

Learning Outcomes: Students will learn how to identify and request library services. Students will understand how to access discipline-specific learning resources. Students will develop basic search strategies using specific databases.

Assessment: At the end of the session, librarians will provide a summative qualitative assessment by asking the students how comfortable they feel with library databases and services.

Activities

Pre-session online tutorial, dialogue about library services and resources, and database exploration.

Activity 1: Students will complete an online tutorial before attending the library's workshop. The self-paced online tutorial illustrates why students need library resources in addition to Google, and how they can best access

Table 5.1. Sample Completet Worksheet

Characteristic	**Observed Qualities of Assigned Source**
Author	Unidentified
Intended audience	Everyone, anyone with RA, anyone who knows someone with RA
Photos/images	One color photo of scientist
Charts/graphs	None
Length of article	Short
Reference list	No references cited

Based on your list of characteristics and observations, what kind of source is this? [*Popular.*]

these resources. Videos and website (screenshot or iFrame) and database information are provided within the tutorial, as well as quick questions students are required to answer. Librarians should identify three or more databases to introduce to their students, as they will use this in the third activity. If access to online tutorial ware is not available, slides with this information and links will also work.

Activity 2—Learning Outcome: Students will understand how to identify and request library services.

1. Librarians should gauge student knowledge of up to five beneficial resources or services for students. Librarians could pull from frequently asked questions at their service desk or questions that surfaced in previous instruction. Ask the students how they approach library services. These questions will start a dialogue with students as they currently understand the library. The students will respond describing the alternatives they use and have available. Librarians should record any points they want to follow up on but allow the dialogue to be conversational and understanding rather than interrupting to highlight any misunderstanding or incorrect information—just let the conversation happen. This dialogue should highlight to the librarian where student knowledge of the library is lacking. Sample questions:

    a. What do you do when you need a space to study?
    b. What do you do when you are not on campus and need help with your research?
    c. What do you do when you need a book, article, or other resource that is not in the library collection?

2. The librarian will present the library's options to satisfy those needs using details and information from the first activity's dialogue. Have a group discussion and contrast the student responses, the problems they encounter, and the options included on the library's website.

Activity 3—Learning Outcome: Students will understand how to access a specific relevant database, and will develop basic search strategies. They can work individually or in small groups of two or three students to explore and describe the outcomes of the following activity to the entire class:

1. Access one of the databases included in the first activity's tutorial. Students should be split evenly among the databases.
2. Select a topic to research and record initial search keyword(s) used in the database.

3. Identify keywords on a topic and where to find synonyms/descriptors/keywords within an article entry.
4. Explore all the possible ways to search for the topic:

    a. Keywords (or free text search)
    b. Subject headings

5. Limit results by date, age group, and/or type of research.
6. Access the full text of an article in the database.
7. Explain how the database could best be used for the research in this class.

Give the various individuals / small groups that searched the same database a few minutes to corroborate or collaborate on what they decide as the best answers. Encourage peer learning.

If your classroom space has an instructor projector / computer space, have each group present on their database to the rest of their class. If your classroom space does not have an instructor projector / computer space, "jig-saw" the students into different groups. For example, students from CINAHL pair with students from Web of Science and PubMed. Have each individual / small group demonstrate to their jig-sawed group. Guide this through limiting time, for example, "Everyone who used CINAHL, you have 4 minutes to demo the database to the rest of your group."

Librarians should refrain from interrupting the student demonstrations but guide students through the process with questions and positive reinforcement (especially if they navigate differently).

Literature Searching to Support Evidence-Based Veterinary Pharmacology

Contributors: Heather K. Moberly, MSLS, FHEA, PgCert (Vet Ed), AHIP (Dorothy G. Whitley Professor, Coordinator of Veterinary Services, Medical Sciences Library, Texas A&M University, College Station); and Sarah K. Bankston, MFA, MSLS (Biomedical Sciences and Veterinary Medicine Librarian, Medical Sciences Library, Texas A&M University, College Station)

Frame—Research as Inquiry. Students are challenged to formulate questions related to specific clinical scenarios using the PICO format. They must identify information gaps and create appropriately scoped searches based on the PICOs to identify published evidence (e.g., articles). They must use the available evidence to make and justify a clinical recommendation for their clinical scenario. Other associated frames: Searching as Strategic Exploration.

Target Audience: Professional veterinary students (DVM/VMD). The session may be adapted for other health sciences disciplines, especially when addressing evidence-based practice.

Setting: This two-hour, hands-on library session is the second week of a 6-week evidence-based veterinary medicine module during Veterinary Pharmacology II for second-year veterinary students. Students develop two PICO questions based on clinical scenarios during week 1 and bring them to the library session. Students use the PICOs to formulate searches for two different databases in order to identify evidence related to the questions. The end products of the 6-week module are treatment recommendations for each of two clinical scenarios and an evidence-based justification for each treatment recommendation.

Learning Outcomes

- **Describe** the subject coverage differences between PubMed and CAB Abstracts related to veterinary medicine.
- **Explain** the circumstances during which you would search each in veterinary medicine.
- **Demonstrate** searching skills in either/both PubMed and CAB Abstracts.
- **Create** an appropriate search strategy using keywords and Boolean logic.

Assessment

The instructor and two librarians "float" during the open searching portion of the session and have one-on-one discussions with students as formative assessment. Students demonstrate their searches and discuss the relevance of the results and next steps to either continue or reconfigure their search. Two one-minute papers allow the students to reflect upon their experiences searching.

Activity

Pre-work:

- Prior to the library session, students are assigned the PubMed for Veterinarians tutorial. http://cases.vetmoodle.org/CET_CoursePlayer/demo1/public/pubmed.html
- Students are instructed to bring two PICO questions from week 1.

Welcome and Introduction: Upon entering class, students either log in to My NCBI or set up an account using directions displayed on the screen. After librarians and instructor welcome the class, students are directed to choose one of their PICO questions and search PubMed for 3–5 minutes. No more specific instruction is provided. This encourages exploration and tests preconceived notions of self-confidence through productive failure.

- Class discusses issues related to search success or failure and appropriateness of results.

Searching Essentials and PubMed: Librarians give a mini-lecture about where to search (library databases) and how to search (generating synonyms and related terms, considering truncation, and developing search strings with Boolean operators). At this point, Google and Google Scholar have intentionally not been addressed.

- Students spend 3–5 minutes brainstorming to revise their search strategy using the best practices discussed in the mini-lecture.

After the students brainstorm and before they return to PubMed to search with their revised strategies, the librarians address the gorilla in the room by giving a mini-lecture about Google Scholar, contrasting its abilities (both positive and negative) with PubMed and library resources.

- Students search PubMed using their newly developed search strategies for 10 minutes, followed by a group discussion of how their results changed.

The librarians review features of PubMed that will help students evaluate their search results and provide search examples from a sample PICO at three different levels of intensity, sophistication, and comprehensiveness.

- Students continue to search for 10 minutes for articles relevant to their PICO. The instructor and librarians discuss results with students on a one-on-one basis.

To finish this section of the session, students write a one-minute paper about the differences between their initial and later stage search results.

CAB Abstracts: The process of searching and readjusting search strategy based on results is repeated with CAB Abstracts. Students write a one-minute paper to reflect on their search results using CAB Abstracts.

Open Searching: For the remainder of the class, the students search using either PubMed or CAB Abstracts, and the instructor and librarians are available to answer questions about the assignment, searching, and results.

- Common questions arise related to not finding enough evidence (e.g., articles) to address their clinical scenarios or finding evidence that is weak. The instructor, librarians, and students discuss strategies for adapting the students' conceptualization of their question and what "evidence" looks like because they are not permitted to adapt their clinical scenario to fit the available evidence. One goal of the overall module is to understand that, regardless of the clinical scenario, as veterinarians they will need to make treatment recommendations.

Wrap-Up: The librarians address common searching issues with the group as a whole. Librarians remind the students about the assistance available outside class time, including e-mail and scheduled appointments. The 6-week module includes two optional sessions, during the scheduled class time, for students to work on the assignment with the librarian available for further assistance.

Aligning Allied Health with ACRL Framework

Contributor: Megan Bell, MLIS (Reference Librarian and Instructor, UAB Libraries, Lister Hill Library of the Health Sciences, University of Alabama at Birmingham)

Frame—Research as Inquiry. Students compare and contrast three locations for retrieving journal articles. Students are encouraged to assess the place in the information search process and match information need with the best resource for that step. Other associated frames: Searching as Strategic Exploration.

Target Audience: Physician assistant (master of science in physician assistant studies) and physical therapy (doctor of physical therapy) students. The lesson may also be adapted to other health sciences disciplines, to include biotechnology, clinical laboratory sciences, genetic counseling, health physics, nuclear medicine technology, occupational therapy, nutrition sciences, and health services administration.

Setting: To be used in a lesson accompanying library instruction for physician assistant students working on systematized review and physical therapy students working on PICO questions.

Learning Outcomes: Students will be able to identify the main ideas of a research question, compare and contrast three locations for searching for articles (library catalog, Google Scholar, and PubMed), and know the advantages and disadvantages of keyword searching. Students will match the search strategy to information need.

Assessment: Open-ended questions used throughout lesson for formative assessment. In addition, students complete a search strategy worksheet for summative assessment.

Activity

Complete aligning of allied health with ACRL Framework either individually or in groups and in person or virtually; however, it needs to be synchronous. Formative assessment resource can use whatever is available.

1. Show sample research question.

    a. Example: Does physical exercise reduce symptoms of ADHD in children?

2. Explain the concept of main ideas and then identify the main ideas in the sample research question.
3. Give a numbered list of sample research questions and allow students to choose one to work through during class.
4. Ask students to write a research question selected on the search strategy worksheet.
5. Ask students to identify main ideas in the question selected.
6. Ask students to put the question number and main idea of the question into live interactive audience participation online software.

    a. Example: #5 exercise ADHD children.

7. Ask students to write the main ideas identified in the table of the search strategy worksheet.
8. Introduce three locations to search for articles (Google Scholar, library catalog, and PubMed). Explain that Google Scholar and library catalog are useful resources when a student is at the beginning of search and wants to do a broad search on topic, but databases are more targeted and useful when a student wants a narrow search.
9. Explain *and*, *or*, *not* are tools used to expand or restrict your search.
10. Ask students to search the library catalog using the main ideas identified on the search strategy worksheet.
11. Ask students to share via live interactive audience participation online software what they notice about the library catalog search.
12. The library catalog searches multiple databases simultaneously. Discuss advantages and disadvantages of searching multiple databases simultaneously.
13. Ask students to search Google Scholar using the main ideas identified on the search strategy worksheet.
14. Compare results and filters of Google Scholar and the library catalog. Ask the class to share two differences via live interactive audience participation online software.

15. Introduce PubMed and explain the concept of a database.
16. Ask students to search PubMed using the main ideas identified on the search strategy worksheet.
17. Explain the advantages and disadvantages of keyword searching in different resources.

Search Strategy Worksheet

Search Question: Write your research question below.

Main Ideas: Examine your research question. What are the main ideas? The chart (see table 5.2) will help you identify some good search terms.

Search Statement: Use the terms from the chart (see table 5.2) to structure a search statement. Use the appropriate connector term (*and*, *or*, *not*).

How many results did you retrieve with the library catalog?
Are the results relevant?
Where is the library catalog searching?
How many results did you retrieve with Google Scholar?
Are the results relevant?
Where is Google Scholar searching?
How many results did you retrieve with PubMed?
Are the results relevant?
Where is PubMed searching?

Reference: Modified from Alverno College Library. (2013). Database search strategy worksheet. Retrieved from http://www.alverno.edu/media/alvernocollege/library/pdfs/DatabaseSearchStrategyWS.pdf

Maximizing Mind Maps: Using Mind Maps to Frame a Research Question and to Develop a Search Strategy

Contributor: Marielle McNeal (Assistant Professor / Head of Teaching and Learning Services, Liaison to the School of Nursing and Health Sciences, Brandel Library, North Park University)

Frame—Research as Inquiry. Other associated frames: Searching as Strategic Exploration.

Table 5.2. Identifying Search Terms

Main Idea	Synonyms and Alternate Ways of Phrasing
1.	
2.	
3.	

Target Audience: Graduate nursing. The lesson may also be adapted for other health disciplines like dentistry, physical/occupational therapy, speech pathology, nutrition, and public health.

Setting: To be used for graduate students that are completing a research-intensive assignment or capstone project. Students in this setting are charged with developing an evidence-based project with the potential for dissemination. Emphasis is placed on framing a well-defined research question.

Time: The total time for this lesson plan is around 90 minutes. Students should come to the session prepared with a broad topic idea.

Learning Outcomes

- Students will recognize the value of building in time to brainstorm their research topics using mind maps.
- Students will be able to narrow a broad topic into a well-defined question that uses the PICO framework.
- Students will be able to identify relevant search terms for their research questions.
- Students will recognize that framing a well-defined research question is intertwined with finding, reading, and analyzing sources.

Assessment

- *Formative:* At the end of the session, students submit a copy of their broad topic, mind map, and a more defined research question that follows the PICO framework.
- *Summative:* A week after the session, students submit a detailed research proposal that includes a well-defined research question that uses the PICO framework, database search terms, and an annotated bibliography (or evidence grid) of supporting evidence.

Materials Needed

- Blank paper
- Colored pencils, pens, or markers
- Instructor computer/projector
- Student computers

The First Step of EBP (5 Minutes)

The librarian displays slides or a short tutorial that emphasizes the following points:

- Brief overview of the five steps of the evidence-based process

- Step 1 of the evidence-based process focuses on framing a well-defined research question.
- Step 1 drives the subsequent steps of the evidence-based process and is key to conducting a quality research project.
- Step 1 is also the most challenging part of the evidence-based process.
- It's important to build in time to brainstorm your research question.

Mind Maps as a Brainstorming Tool (5 Minutes)

The librarian displays several examples of mind maps and emphasizes the following points:

- Mind mapping is the process of taking a broad topic and visually breaking it down into smaller topics.
- Mind mapping allows you to find connections between concepts/topics.
- Mind mapping can help you find a manageable area of study and develop a well-defined research question.

Mind Mapping Activity (30 Minutes)

Students are provided time to create their own mind maps on paper or using free websites like Coggle.it, Mindmeister, Bubbl.us, MindMup, among others. The librarian and teaching faculty observe and offer guidance to students that need additional help.

Students are prompted to address the following guiding questions in their mind maps:

- What population or patient group are you interested in? What are the most important characteristics (age, gender, race, etc.) of the population or patient group?
- What main interventions are you considering? What do you want to do with this population or patient group?
- What are the main alternative treatments that you are considering, if any?
- What are you hoping to accomplish, measure, improve, or effect?

PICO Framework and Question Types (10 Minutes)

The librarian displays several examples of well-defined research questions that use the PICO framework and provides a handout with a description of the four question types. The following points are emphasized:

- The guiding questions from the mind map activity are based on the PICO framework.

- PICO is a mnemonic used to describe the four important elements of a well-defined research question.
- PICO elements change according to the question type (therapy, prevention, diagnosis, prognosis, and etiology).
- Identifying your PICO elements is essential for developing an effective search strategy.

Identifying PICO Elements Activity (5 Minutes)

Students use colored pencils, pens, or markers to identify the PICO elements in their mind maps.

Research Questions and Search Terms Activity (15 Minutes)

Students are provided time to create a draft of a well-defined research question that uses the PICO framework. Students will then use their PICO elements to develop database search terms (see table 5.3).

Broad topic that you started with:
More defined research question:
Question type:
PICO elements and database search terms (don't forget about CINAHL Headings/MeSH):

Finding Relevant Evidence Activity (20 Minutes)

The librarian demonstrates a sample search in CINAHL or a related health sciences database. Students will spend the remainder of the session finding, reading, and analyzing sources that are relevant to their research question.

After spending some time reviewing relevant evidence, how might you revise your research question?

Review and Wrap Up (5 Minutes)

Students are encouraged to continue searching and reading sources after the workshop. The librarian should emphasize that developing a well-defined research question is intertwined with reading and analyzing sources. If time

Table 5.3. PICO Elements and Database Search Terms

	Population	Intervention	Comparison	Outcome
PICO Elements				
Search Terms				
Headings/MeSH				

permits, a follow-up lesson or workshop should be provided to teach students how to read and analyze evidence-based research articles.

Framing the Clinical Question: From Topic Idea to PICO

Contributor: Stephanie Debner, MA, MLIS (Head of Library Public Services [Reference, Instruction & Access Services], W. A. Budden Library, University of Western States)

Frame—Research as Inquiry. Students learn to formulate appropriate clinical questions and break them down into researchable components. Through the process of forming a well-constructed PICO, students are prompted to ask more complex questions through further inquiry by narrowing down the topic scope and choosing relevant search terms. Organizing information by clinical category types also helps students limit the scope of their investigations and organize information in meaningful ways. Other associated frames: Searching as Strategic Exploration.

Target Audience: Postgraduate/professional students in chiropractic. The lesson may also be adapted to all other health sciences disciplines with an evidence-based practice focus.

Setting: Used with postgraduate/professional chiropractic students in one class session of a term-long, hybrid introductory course on evidence-based practice (EBP) and searching research literature. Over the term, students are expected to master the foundational concepts of EBP and apply strategies in the information search process. The lesson presumes that students have working knowledge of clinical categories and PICO and have had exposure to well-designed clinical questions. It is designed for the classroom but could be adapted for online instruction.

Learning Outcomes: Students will identify clinical questions by category (therapy, diagnosis, harm, prognosis). Students will break up different kinds of clinical questions into PICO elements. Students will translate topics from basic topic statements in nonclinical language into discipline-relevant clinical questions.

Assessment: With the clinical category notecard activity, the different colors make it quick and easy to assess student responses and address gaps in understanding. Padlet activity can be used as graded item to assess student skill in writing clinical questions, attributing questions to the correct clinical category, and extracting PICO elements from clinical questions.

Activity: Clinical Questions, Categories, and PICO Activity

Completed in class either individually or in small groups; could be adapted to be completed independently or online outside of the classroom. The instructor projects slides with activity elements; students also have access to slides online. The activity presumes that students (individually or per small group) have a computer, laptop, or tablet.

Part 1: Students are given four discipline-relevant clinical questions on handout(s) and four different colored notecards with the clinical categories written on them (therapy, diagnosis, harm, prognosis).

a. As each question is projected on-screen, students hold up the colored card with the category they think matches the question.
b. Follow with a quick discussion for any differences observed in student responses; if needed, point out clues in the questions that point to the clinical category.
c. Students circle and label PICO elements in the clinical questions.
d. Follow-up: the whole class reviews questions together (projected on-screen) with student volunteers providing PICO elements; the instructor fills in PICO elements on slides based on student input.

Examples of clinical questions for Part 1:

- For patients with Achilles tendon rupture, is conservative care effective in shortening return to sport compared to surgery?
- Is participation in gymnastics a risk factor for spondylolisthesis?
- Compared to MRI, is ultrasound accurate in detecting a partial rupture of the Achilles tendon?
- How does a sedentary lifestyle versus an active lifestyle influence the resolution of low back pain?

Part 2: Students choose one of four provided topics worded in nonclinical language. Note: students will likely have to add information to the topics to make a fully rounded clinical question.

a. Reword the topic as a discipline-appropriate clinical question, identify the clinical category the question belongs to, and break the question into PICO elements.
b. Post the question, clinical category, and PICO to the Padlet page for this activity.
c. The instructor pulls up Padlet on classroom screen to show student posts in real time.
d. Follow-up: whole class discussion of choices made in clinical questions, clinical category assignments, and PICO breakdowns.

Examples of topics for Part 2:

- Group exercise is better for older adults than individual workouts.
- Yoga is more dangerous than you think.
- Tai chi is good for cardiac rehabilitation.
- Ultrasound is the best way to diagnose shoulder injuries.

Chapter Six

Scholarship as Conversation

This frame asserts that the scholarly discourse surrounding a topic is an ongoing conversation into which new authors enter. Using this analogy helps students understand the importance of conducting thorough literature reviews in order to capture relevant contributions to this conversation. Similarly, it also reinforces the importance of citing their referenced materials.

Not all conversations are peaceful, though, and this extends into scholarly conversation as well. It is important for students to recognize that diverging viewpoints can be found within many research topics. Effective literature reviews should highlight main camps and lead voices representing different sides of debates. It is important for students to learn to at least nod to viewpoints that differ from their own, even if only to proceed to refute them with new or alternative evidence. Emerging scholars need assistance in this process. Librarians can hold a pivotal role in teaching literature review design that reveals diverging viewpoints and does not simply achieve confirmation bias.

A didactic approach that is highly valued in current health sciences education is interprofessional education, or IPE. IPE can be built into the curriculum, the clinical experiences, and the very physical spaces of health sciences educational programs. How fitting that it is considered a research strategy as well. Akin to the more widely recognized interdisciplinary education, IPE intentionally mimics patient-centered care models in which a patient is positioned at the center, with a care team circled around them to achieve dynamic, informed, and collaborative care with the patient's needs and preferences in mind. An IPE teaching module might pair a medical student to provide medical recommendations with a social work student to advise on the patient's cognitive ability to take medicine on a schedule and their mobility/access to transportation in order to attend physical therapy as prescribed.

Librarians engaged with health sciences programs that incorporate IPE concepts can integrate IPE into search strategies in a couple of different ways. One approach is to run consecutive searches in a variety of discipline-specific databases to see how professionals in each field address the issue. This can help students identify the potential roles that members of a care team can fill and the expertise they can provide for a specific health concern or treatment approach. This approach can prove to be time-consuming but can be streamlined thanks to the utilization of the National Library of Medicine's controlled health sciences vocabulary—Medical Subject Headings, or MeSH—by numerous health sciences databases: once effective keywords or subject terms are identified, they can be used successfully across many databases.

An alternative approach to uncover interprofessional literature is to run the search in a database that indexes articles from numerous disciplines. There are many databases and journal collections designed to operate in this manner, including licensed and open access. Health sciences researchers can benefit from going a step beyond the expected and turning to a wider variety of databases that lie outside of the traditional health sciences titles. A nursing student seeking information on the best way to staff a hospital floor during a nursing shortage might find relevant articles in the nursing literature, health care administration literature, business/human resources literature, and even psychology literature addressing employee burnout and strategies to prevent it. Health sciences students who learn to leverage evidence and effective strategies from professionals in all domains will bring creative solutions to their future career fields; librarians are poised to teach them how to find evidence to inspire and to support their innovative strategies.

Undergraduate research classes in most disciplines call for students to identify voices in the scholarly conversation that carry the most weight. These voices can hold esteem for a number of reasons, for example, pioneers in the field, current innovators in the given field, and researchers affiliated with respected programs in the field. Students need to be taught how to identify these voices when conducting literature searches via strategies such as citation tracking, performing author searches in databases, and the tried-and-true method of reading numerous articles and noticing the same figures referenced repeatedly.

Once students understand this concept and have identified these leading voices, teaching faculty and librarians can take the discussion one step further and have students consider why these voices are so prominent, which voices tend to rise to the top, and which voices are underrepresented. Termed critical information literacy, this approach calls on researchers to acknowledge power structures at play behind the voices that emerge—and those that don't—in the scholarly discourse. All disciplines have hierarchies of scholars, including the health sciences, which are driven by politics, funding, and powerful publishing houses. As students progress through their academic tenure, they should be made aware of the power dynamics that lead to the literature that sits before them.

Scholarship as Conversation is such a relatable, teachable concept across disciplines and student levels. It is nowhere more relevant than in the cutthroat publishing environment present in the health sciences. Librarians working with this population can equip the next generation with the tools and strategies required to learn from the past while envisioning the future.

SCHOLARSHIP AS CONVERSATION IN ACTION: CASE STUDIES

Framing Library Instruction for Evidence-Based Public Health

Contributor: Leah Cordova, MLIS (Assistant Professor at the University of Tennessee Health Science Center and Research & Learning Services Librarian at the university's Health Sciences Library)

Frame—Scholarship as Conversation. Other associated frames: Information Creation as a Process and Searching as Strategic Exploration.

Target Audience: Undergraduate public health students. The lesson may also be adapted for health sciences disciplines, to include pre-professional/professional health students.

Setting: Public health students are enrolled in a semester-long health information research course, co-taught with departmental faculty and a librarian. Students are asked to research a specific health issue/disparity over the course of the semester. By this point, students have already identified the health issue of interest as well as the population most impacted by the health issue. For this particular assignment, students are asked to identify public health intervention(s) that could be used to address this health issue given their specific population, keeping in mind concepts of evidence-based public health practice.

Learning Outcomes: Students will be able to articulate the concept of evidence-based practice as it pertains to public health in order to demonstrate an understanding of the value of research in the field. Students will be able to construct effective and iterative searches in appropriate search tools, to find relevant interventions given their health issue and population.

Assessment: Formative assessment in the form of in-class discussion and a summative assessment of student learning with a worksheet are included in this lesson.

Conversation at a Glance: Quick Tips for Busy Librarians

Scholarship as Conversation

Communities of scholars, researchers, or professionals engage in sustained discourse with new insights and discoveries occurring over time as a result of varied perspectives and interpretations.

http://www.ala.org/acrl/standards/ilframework

Pedagogical Point: Discursive
"Research in scholarly and professional fields is a discursive practice in which ideas are formulated, debated, and weighed against one another over extended periods of time." (Framework)

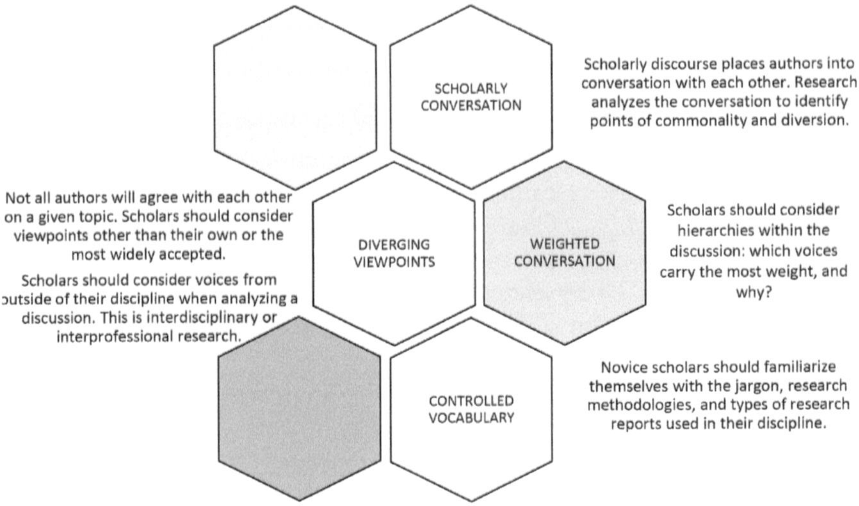

Special considerations for the health sciences:

- ❑ Scholars are never too inexperienced to join the conversation. Health sciences students enter the scholarly discussion when they write and present within their classes and programs.

FRAMING HEALTHCARE 5

Activity

Step 1. Pre-class Readings: Before class, students are asked to review the following articles. Below each of the articles are the main concepts students are asked to consider during their review.

1. Jacobs, J. A., Jones, E., Gabella, B. A., Spring, B., & Brownson, R. C. (2012). Tools for implementing an evidence-based approach in public health practice. *Preventing Chronic Disease*, 9. Retrieved from https://doi.org/10.5888/pcd9.110324

    a. What are the main ideas or concepts behind evidence-based public health?
    b. Why is there a need for evidence-based public health practice?

2. Green, L. W. (2008). Making research relevant: If it is an evidence-based practice, where's the practice-based evidence? *Family Practice,* 25, i20–i24. Retrieved from https://doi.org/10.1093/fampra/cmn055

    a. What does the author mean by a "pipeline" of transferring research to practice?
    b. What are some of the main issues with this "pipeline" concept?
    c. What information or whose voices might not be represented in this "pipeline"?
    d. What strategies does the author suggest could improve the flow of information through the "pipeline"?

Step 2. Evidence-Based Public Health Practice Classroom Discussion

1. Reading Review

    a. In-class discussion regarding main concepts of the two articles. Students are asked to articulate main concepts of evidence-based practice, how this applies to public health, and why it is necessary. Furthermore, students discuss issues regarding the "pipeline" of transferring research into practice and whose voices may not be being heard but could still be valuable. Students' understandings of these concepts serve as a formative assessment of main ideas.

2. Resources Introduction and Overview

    a. Students are introduced to various resources they can use to find evidence-based public health interventions, such as the Community Guide and evidence-based search features in PubMed.

Step 3. Class Activity and Homework

Consider the Evidence

In class today, we went over several resources you can use to find literature on public health interventions. For this exercise, you will need to use one or more of those resources to locate an intervention you could potentially implement to address your health issue. Keep in mind that you may not be able to find an intervention that pertains both to your specific population and your specific health issue. Sometimes you need to consult multiple interventions that you could mesh together to implement something for your population's specific need.

- What information resource(s) did you use to find intervention(s)?
- What health issue is addressed through the intervention(s)? This should be your health topic; if it is not you will need to be able to make the case as to why you chose this intervention and how this approach could be utilized for your health issue given your population.
- What are the objectives of selected intervention(s), or what were they hoping to accomplish?
- Did they consider their intervention to be successful? Why or why not?
- What population does your selected intervention(s) serve?
- Is the population the same as the population you are researching? (yes/no)
- If no, are there any similarities between the population you are studying and the population the intervention focuses on? Please explain.
- How does identifying an established public health intervention fit in with the concept of evidence-based practice?
- Why is it valuable to identify existing public health interventions before implementing your own?

Evidence-Based Practice in Nursing Pharmacology: Herbal Supplements and Clinical Decision Making

Contributors: Kristi Coe, MS, RN, MLIS student (Health Sciences Librarian, Cedarville University); and Angelia Mickle, DNP, RN, APRN, FNP-C, CEN (Dean, School of Nursing, Cedarville University)

Frame—Research as Inquiry. Research is iterative and depends upon asking increasingly complex or new questions whose answers in turn develop additional questions or lines of inquiry in any field (object 1 and object 3).

Frame—Scholarship as Conversation. Communities of scholars, researchers, or professionals engage in sustained discourse with new insights and discoveries occurring over time as a result of varied perspectives and interpretations (object 2).

Target Audience: Undergraduate, second-year nursing (could be adapted to undergraduate pre-pharmacy or allied health).

Setting: Lesson given spring semester of the sophomore year to BSN students in NSG 3110: Pharmacology subsequent to IL/library introduction through both First-Year Instruction program and discipline-specific instruction in the freshman year.

Learning Outcomes

- Objective 1: Demonstrate an introductory understanding of evidence-based practice including PICO questions format ***(Research as Inquiry)***
- Objective 2: Demonstrate proficiency with a variety of library and publicly available resources to answer a clinical question ***(Scholarship as Conversation)***
- Objective 3: Apply class content on herbal supplements to a clinical problem using best evidence ***(Research as Inquiry)***

Activity—Research and Group Presentation: The health sciences librarian (HSL) will provide an overview of evidence-based research methods for students. Specific topics will be assigned to student groups of four or five. Specifics regarding the assignment and rubric are available in the learning management system (LMS). Following your exploration for best practice guidelines, groups will provide a creative information sharing presentation during the seminar. Each presentation will be roughly 8–10 minutes. Everyone is expected to demonstrate participation.

Lesson Plan for a 75-Minute Class

General Overview by HSL: Reintroduction/Library Website (10 minutes)

- Reminder of purpose of HSL
- Library website review: how to get to website; key features: OneSearch, individual databases, library catalog; research guides (PICOT)

OneSearch Review (10 minutes)

- Purpose
- Spectrum of search
- Limiters
- Controlled vocabulary

What if I can't get to my article or still have questions? (5 minutes)

- ILL

- Research appointment

Assignment-Specific Instruction by HSL

- Work through PICO tutorial on PubMed covering MeSH and searching strategies (https://www.youtube.com/watch?v=_pVxRw-y8-M&t=36s) (15 minutes).
- Clinical databases (including LexiComp and UpToDate) and NIH sites as supplemental information (10 minutes).

Work Groups (HSL and Teaching Faculty):

- Work on completing assignment to help prepare for presentation. HSL and teaching faculty will circulate and answer individual/group questions (20 minutes).

Pharmacology Research Assignment Worksheet

1. Name the herbal supplement that has been assigned to your group:
2. Develop a PICO question based on your assigned topic.
3. Use OneSearch to conduct an initial query (adjust your PICO based on results if needed).

    - Search terms used:
    - Number of initial results:
    - Limiters applied:

4. Choose a database (PubMed, CINAHL, or Medline is recommended) and use their controlled vocabulary options to identify alternate search terms (i.e., hypericum for St. John's Wort). List alternate terms:
5. Find three scholarly resources that will help answer the following questions:

    - Purported uses of herbal supplement
    - Supporting evidence for use
    - Drug interactions
    - Potential adverse effects
    - Your group's recommendation for use of the herbal supplement

6. Search a clinical database such as 1) LexiComp or 2) UpToDate or a publicly available resource such as 3) National Center for Complementary and Integrative Health (NIH) to see if any additional information should be added to your final recommendation. Compare and

contrast with information found in the databases. List any additional information below:

Assessment Rubric—Pharmacology Research Assignment Grading Rubric

Group Name:
Students:

1. Develop a PICO question based on your assigned topic (25 points)
2. Identify database used and three scholarly resources (25 points)
3. Presentation includes: (50 points; 10 for each category)

- Purported uses of herbal supplement
- Supporting evidence for use
- Drug interactions
- Potential adverse effects
- Your group's recommendation for use of the herbal supplement

Graduate-Level Research in an Online Nursing Program: From Novice to Expert

Contributor: Kyle Lynes, MLIS (Reference Librarian, Mortensen Library, University of Hartford)

Frame—Scholarship as Conversation. Online graduate nursing students access a suite of online tools in lieu of face-to-face instruction. Both before and after working through an interactive tutorial and viewing short screencasts, students take a quiz.

Other associated frames: Authority Is Constructed and Contextual, Research as Inquiry, and Searching as Strategic Exploration.

Target Audience: Graduate nursing (MSN). These resources may also be adapted to other health sciences disciplines.

Setting: Library instruction modules have been created for two online graduate nursing courses. Both modules are accessed virtually by students prior to starting a research project. Embedded into the online introductory MSN course, the first module acts as a research refresher for first-semester students. Embedded into a research-intensive MSN course, the second module covers advanced research in the health sciences in preparation for a literature review.

Learning Outcomes: After completing the introductory module, students will better understand basic research theory and its practical application within the health sciences. Completion of the advanced module will better prepare students to conduct high-level research. Both modules will give students exposure to library resources and services.

Assessment: Students take a 20-question pretest before the modules are released. The test is taken again after students have worked through the content. All questions are directly related to the content covered within the modules, with the exception of two questions designed to gauge students' attitudes toward research.

Library Instruction Modules

Both library instruction modules contain three components: an interactive tutorial, several short screencasts, and a nursing LibGuide.

Tutorials: Interactive tutorials were created using PowerPoint and i-Spring Suite. The tutorials are hosted on the library's server and embedded directly into the course shell. The introductory tutorial covers the following content:

- Planning stages of research: defining a topic and research statement, establishing key concepts and search terms, finding synonyms, and narrowing/expanding a topic.
- Article types: peer review, primary versus secondary research articles, types of articles within the health sciences, and the anatomy of an article.
- Database searching: CINAHL versus ProQuest Nursing and Allied Health, keyword searching, advanced search page features, results page features, and accessing articles.
- Evaluating websites: types of websites and evaluation criteria.
- Citing sources: importance of citations, when to cite, in-text and reference list citations, the anatomy of an APA citation for a journal article, and citation resources.

Designed to prepare students to write a literature review, the two-part advanced tutorial covers the following content:

- Advanced searching: Boolean operators, search syntax (phrase searching, truncation, and wildcard searching), narrowing/expanding a topic, and creating a search string.
- Article types: qualitative versus quantitative research, experimental and observational studies, and secondary research.
- Peer review: peer review defined, and why peer-reviewed articles are used.
- Research as a conversation: scholarly conversation defined, entering the conversation, citation chasing, and cited reference searching.
- Literature reviews: literature review defined, categories of literature reviews, and the steps of writing a literature review.

- Ethics and the Institutional Review Board (IRB): ethical issues in research, IRB—what it is and how it works.
- Citing sources: importance of citations, when to cite, in-text and reference list citations, the anatomy of an APA citation for a journal article, and citation resources.

Screencasts: Several short screencasts were recorded to offer live demonstration of library databases, resources, and services. Each screencast was recorded in Camtasia and then uploaded to Ensemble (the university's streaming media server). Captions were added to each screencast using the captioning tool within Ensemble. Most of the screencasts are less than 5 minutes long. The introductory library instruction module contains four screencasts:

- Overview of the library website: top tools, library chat, accessing the OPAC, accessing databases, and the Interlibrary Loan portal.
- Searching in CINAHL: advanced search with basic filters, results page features, full text versus non–full text results, the detailed record, and useful tools at the article level.
- Searching in ProQuest Nursing and Allied Health Source: advanced search page with basic filters, results page features, full text versus non–full text results, the detailed record, and useful tools at the article level.
- Interlibrary Loan: creating an account, requesting materials, and accessing materials.

The advanced library instruction module contains three screencasts:

- Advanced searching in databases: proper use of Boolean operators, application of search syntax, inputting a complex search string.
- Specialty database filters: first or any author is a nurse, population filters, research study type, setting.
- Using our journal finder tool: how to check coverage of a specific journal title within our electronic and print holdings.

Nursing LibGuide: Both modules also contain links to our nursing LibGuide, which contains a carefully curated list of resources in the following categories:

- Books
- Specific journal titles
- Databases related to the health sciences
- Websites

- Overview of the research process
- Working with APA citations

Role of Systematic Reviews in Evidence-Based Practice

Contributor: Hannah Schilperoort, MLIS, MA (Information Services Librarian, Norris Medical Library, University of Southern California)

Frame—Scholarship as Conversation. Students engage in discourse about the role of systematic reviews and evidence synthesis in evidence-based practice. Students are challenged to identify systematic review methodologies and critically evaluate the quality of published systematic reviews.

Other associated frames: Authority Is Constructed and Contextual and Information Creation as Process.

Target Audience: Graduate nursing (MSN, PHD, DNP). The lesson may also be adapted to other health sciences disciplines, including graduate medical, pharmacy, dental, occupational therapy, physical therapy, and other allied health degrees.

Setting: To be used with graduate nursing students in an evidence-based practice or research methods course in preparation for the final paper. Students are charged with finding multiple types of high-level sources published within the last 5 years to answer a PICOT question. Students must critically appraise each source as well as combine and contrast findings to form conclusions based on the overall evidence.

Earlier in the course, students receive instruction on database keyword and subject searching and levels of evidence for evidence-based practice. Prior to the activities in this lesson plan, students receive instruction on the definition and role of systematic reviews and research synthesis in evidence-based practice. In an online course, students may receive this instruction asynchronously prior to the live virtual class session. In an on-campus course, students may receive instruction in previous class sessions or at the very beginning of this class session.

Learning Outcomes: Students will be able to:

1. recognize a correct definition of the term *systematic review*;
2. differentiate between a literature review and a systematic review based on the stated review methodologies in the published manuscript; and
3. evaluate the quality of a published systematic review using the Joanna Briggs Institute (JBI) critical appraisal checklist for systematic reviews.

Assessment—Poll Question: Ask the poll question at the beginning of the session to ensure that the librarian, faculty, and students are working with the same shared definition. Another variation of this question would also work.

What is a systematic review? Choose all that apply.

a. A type of high-level evidence synthesis.
b. Answers a specific clinical question by analyzing published and unpublished results from all relevant studies on a given topic.
c. Follows a set of clearly specified, rigorous, reproducible, and transparent methods.
d. Summarizes evidence on a topic using informal or subjective methods to collect and interpret studies.
e. Identifies, selects, and summarizes findings of available research to make clear what is known—and still not known—about a topic.

Correct answer: A, B, C, and E; incorrect answer: D.

Activity 1: Differentiate between a systematic review and a literature review. Students are given a systematic review and a literature review to examine. Remove the title and abstract from each review. Students work in pairs or small groups to compare and contrast the published manuscripts, especially the "Methods" section, to differentiate between the systematic review and the literature review. Each group may be assigned their own unique set of reviews, or all groups may be assigned the same two reviews. Students report their findings to the class for feedback from the librarian, nursing faculty, and fellow students. Each group answers the following questions about each review:

a. Is this a systematic review or a literature review?
b. What details from the manuscript led you to this conclusion?

Activity 2: Evaluate the quality of a published systematic review using the JBI critical appraisal checklist for systematic reviews. Critical appraisal checklists created by other organizations, such as the Critical Appraisal Skills Program (CASP) or Centre for Evidence-Based Medicine (CEBM), may be used in place of the JBI checklist.

Students work in pairs or groups to critically appraise a systematic review using the JBI checklist. Each group may critically appraise a different systematic review, or each group may be assigned a section of the checklist for a single systematic review. Students present their appraisals to the class for feedback from the librarian, nursing faculty, and fellow students.

The checklist is publicly available on the JBI website. Create a table based on the checklist on a Google Doc or other cloud-based collaborative tool for student collaboration online or in person.

See table 6.1 for an example of how to construct a table based on the JBI critical appraisal checklist for systematic reviews.

Gearing up for Grand Rounds

Contributors: Fiona Inglis, MI, MA (Librarian, Centre for Addiction & Mental Health, Toronto, Canada); and Sharon Bailey, MI, AHIP (Manager, Library & Archives, Centre for Addiction & Mental Health, Toronto, Canada)

Frame—Scholarship as Conversation. Other associated frames: Research as Inquiry, Searching as Strategic Exploration.

Target Audience: Psychiatry residents.

Setting: The Centre for Addiction & Mental Health is a teaching hospital affiliated with the University of Toronto. Psychiatry residents are required to present a Grand Round once each academic year. Topics are chosen by the residents. This workshop is designed to help the residents develop an effective search strategy for the literature review component of their presentation. Because the Grand Rounds are scheduled throughout the year, not all participants will have a topic in mind when they take this workshop. It is held in a computer lab and usually has 10 participants.

Learning Outcomes: By the end of this workshop participants will be able to:

- discuss the role that Grand Rounds play in the scholarly conversation;
- explore a range of perspectives within the scholarly conversation;
- evaluate their current strategies for participating in the scholarly conversation; and
- develop, document, and share effective search strategies.

Table 6.1. Critical Appraisal

	Yes	No	Unclear	Not Applicable	Reasons for Your Decision and Sections in the Article Where You Found the Evidence
1. Is the review question clearly and explicitly stated?					

Assessment

Formative: Completion of the workshop activities.

Summative: Performance in the Grand Round as assessed by both professors and peers using a rubric developed by the Department of Psychiatry.

Activity

Opening Discussion

What are Grand Rounds? Why do we have them? What is your experience of them? Do you have any concerns about presenting one?

Reflecting on Grand Rounds: Use two paragraphs, one describing a slightly negative example of a Grand Round and the other describing what a perfect Grand Round could look like (e.g., excerpts from Ali, S. K., & Saikumar, H. (2015). Not so grand rounds. *Journal of Graduate Medical Education , 7*(2), 304–305. Give one half of the group the positive paragraph and the other the negative paragraph and ask them to read. After a couple of minutes reading, they pair up with someone who read a different paragraph and work together to complete the table presented in table 6.2.

Have a brief discussion to share and summarize findings. Ensure that the role of the patient is covered in the discussion.

Exploring the Evidence: Show whatever form of the evidence-based pyramid you like to work with and lead a discussion on problems with this model from the perspective of Scholarship as Conversation. Topics to include:

- Whose voice is included, and whose is excluded? (e.g., patient and family perspectives)
- Who has access to these resources, and who doesn't? (e.g., patients or rural health professionals without university or hospital libraries)
- What are the specific mental health and addictions research challenges? (e.g., the lack of RCTs on some topics due to vulnerable populations, or new and emerging topics with a limited evidence base)

Planning Your Search: Provide the group with a choice of three scenarios designed to reflect the kinds of situations that might provide the basis for a Grand Rounds topic. Examples include a clinical case study that prompts questions about patient care, a recent health-related news or magazine article

Table 6.2. Grand Round Comparison Exercise

Problems Discussed in the Article	Solutions Suggested in the Article	Your Opinion

that they want to verify, or a trend that they observe in practice and want to explore the evidence surrounding it.

Ask participants to work in pairs and brainstorm the questions they would have about this scenario. Remind them to consider all aspects, including biological, psychological, and social.

Share the questions as a group and then ask them to choose one question and fill in the worksheet (table 6.3).

Ask the whole group to discuss their ideas and think about how to balance reliable evidence with inclusion of all relevant voices.

Searching the Literature: Demonstrate and provide instruction on how to search the resources of your choice. Make sure you include a grey literature component as well as a medical database. Participants can search on their topic and fill in the following fields:

- Main concepts
- Subject headings
- Keywords
- Limits

Documenting Your Search: Ask participants to look at the description of a search strategy provided, for example, in the following article: Shen, N., Sockalingam, S., Abi Jaoude, A., et al. (2017). Scoping review protocol: Education initiatives for medical psychiatry collaborative care. *BMJ Open, 7*(9). doi:10.1136/bmjopen-2017-015886

Ask participants to fill in the blanks with the information from the article:

- Databases
- Search terms
- Search limits
- Other information

Participants should think about describing their search strategy during their Grand Round. Use the following prompts:

Table 6.3. Grand Round Brainstorming Worksheet

Research Question:

Concept	**Search Terms**	**Perspectives**	**Places**
List the concepts your question covers. Think about the problem, the population, interventions, outcomes.	*For each concept think of the words that are used to talk about it.*	*Who would have an interest or an opinion on this concept?*	*Where are the best places to look for information about this topic?*

- How much detail will you need?
- Which pieces of information are the most important?
- Is there anything else you would include that was not mentioned in the example?

Participants can then use the search template provided for Grand Rounds and take it in turns to present their search process to the group.

Summarize and Evaluate: Summarize the main points covered and ask participants to submit their workshop evaluation forms.

Chapter Seven

Searching as Strategic Exploration

Strategic exploration. Experienced researchers will nod their heads knowingly at this descriptive label for the research process. *Exploration* because a question is asked, but the expected answer is not guaranteed. The literature can surprise us with its answers and challenge our assumptions. *Strategic* because while a researcher cannot control their search results, they can help keep the search process focused on the end goal by using proven search tools and techniques.

A reasonable set of learning outcomes that can be extrapolated from the knowledge practices and learner dispositions for this frame include the following:

- **Determine** information need
- **Develop** a research question
- **Identify** sources of information
- **Employ** effective search strategies
- **Utilize** controlled vocabulary
- **Analyze** search results
- **Modify** subsequent searches

When viewed in light of Bloom's Taxonomy (referenced in chapter 3), the verbs listed above are strong and represent a wide range of proficiencies that are applicable to entry-level students and professional researchers alike. Each of these proficiencies is discussed below within the context of health sciences research.

DETERMINE INFORMATION NEED

In order to perform an effective search for information, the searcher must have a clear goal in mind. Health sciences research goals are often very specific and build on the efforts of those who have gone before in a given field. Previous research performed on a topic might have yielded inconclusive results. Alternatively, research might have pointed to an answer previously; however, knowledge has since changed, and the process bears repeating and updating. And, excitingly, medical professionals are pioneering new ideas and techniques all the time that need to be brought to life through testing and trials.

The student populations that we are addressing in this handbook will have varying research needs based on their maturity in the field. Undergraduate health sciences students might be assigned a topic for research, or given a list from which to select. Librarians can assist them in developing search strategies, but the students might not have flexibility to adjust their research questions without the approval of their professor. Graduate health sciences students may be enrolled in clinical experiences that direct their research interests and questions. At both the undergraduate and graduate level, the end goal is often a completed assignment rather than eventual contribution to the scholarly discourse in their discipline. These types of inquiry offer student researchers opportunities to practice and hone their research skills for future application.

The research needs of residents and practicing health professionals will differ from those of health sciences students. The focus shifts from grades and finding a topic the professor will accept to tenure and pursuing a research question for which the academy needs an answer. These researchers can be much more focused in their information-seeking process and will seek less affirmation on project direction from assisting librarians. There will be genres of research within this population, however, for which librarians may be heavily consulted regarding project feasibility and scope (e.g., systematic reviews).

An aspect of determining information need that can be relevant to researchers of all levels is adherence to standards set by governing institutional and federal bodies such as Institutional Review Boards (IRBs), Institutional Animal Care and Use Committees (IACUCs), and grant-finding agencies such as the National Institutes of Health (NIH). Applications for governing committees and grant-funding agencies often have very specific literature review and/or "alternatives to use" components that help demonstrate the need for such research, the value and necessity of any testing done on humans or animals, and the justification of grant monies to carry out the research.

DEVELOP A RESEARCH QUESTION

Once the scope and type of needed information have been clearly identified, the health sciences researcher needs to develop a tailored research question. Health sciences research methodologies will often mirror those in other disciplines; for example, population study research questions may look similar in both a public health class and a more liberal arts–based psychology class. Descriptive, causal, and case studies are examples of methodologies that can cross disciplinary borders.

Health sciences professionals seeking information in a clinical setting will sometimes turn to a question type designed for maximum efficiency: the PICO(T) question. PICO(T) questions are designed to provide busy clinicians with a construct that helps organize the moving parts of their information need.

P = population or patient
I = intervention
C = comparison
O = outcome
(T) = time; not always relevant

Students learning to search for clinical information are sometimes given assignments based around the formulation and answering of a PICO(T) question, whereas practicing clinicians might reflexively fill in the letters of the acronym in the natural course of their thinking about the question at hand. An example PICO(T) question is provided below:

- In pediatric patients with severe peanut allergies, (Population)
- does oral immunotherapy (Intervention)
- in the first five years of life (Time frame)
- yield decreased severity in allergic responses (Outcome)
- as opposed to no treatment? (Comparison)

Based on the above PICO(T) question, a search strategy might be organized thusly in a database:

KW: peanut allergy
KW: oral immunotherapy
KW: outcomes

The researcher could refine the results to pediatric population by including it as a fourth keyword, adding a population-based limit if available in the database selected, or by analyzing each article for applicability.

IDENTIFY DATABASES / INFORMATION SOURCES

Armed with a clearly defined information need and a carefully drafted research question, health sciences researchers can turn to a wide variety of information sources to answer their research questions. Licensed databases aimed at health sciences populations abound. There are databases that are specialty specific and databases that are interprofessional in nature and combine research from multiple medical and allied health specialties. They offer researchers access to search features such as limits relating to the patient population or the clinical setting in question, such as pediatric or adolescent and male or female, and inpatient or outpatient.

Some libraries offer a federated search overlay that sits on top of their collection like an umbrella. Discipline-specific limits are often lost in these federated searches, but the opportunity to perform comprehensive, interdisciplinary searches is gained. Researchers can be surprised where the answer to their research question might live. Rather than knowing on the front end the stake that varying disciplines all hold in the discussion, a federated search allows the researcher to simply ask their question and then discover disciplines that might help provide an answer.

For researchers who are not affiliated with an academic or hospital library, there are numerous open access avenues they can pursue to discover and secure literature. A freely available starting point for health sciences research and literature is PubMed (https://www.ncbi.nlm.nih.gov/pubmed/). Much of the information located in the many NIH, National Library of Medicine (NLM), and National Center for Biotechnology Information (NCBI) databases is open access. For peer-reviewed articles that are located behind publisher paywalls, researchers can use free databases for discovery and then initiate interlibrary loan requests through their public library, or opt to pay the single-article fee for immediate access. And, the unaffiliated researcher will find access to numerous journals that are open access and freely readable. Many authors deposit full-text articles in institutional repositories. Additionally, federal regulations passed in 2013 required that the results of research funded by a set level of federal funding must be available to the public who supported it with their tax dollars; consequently, some articles published in licensed journals can also be freely accessible to the public (see Expanding Public Access to the Results of Federally Funded Research: https://obamawhitehouse.archives.gov/blog/2013/02/22/expanding-public-access-results-federally-funded-research).

A specialized form of health sciences research is the search for evidence-based practice (EBP) resources. When a researcher asks a librarian to help locate evidence to answer their question or to support their position, a good first step for the librarian is to establish a shared understanding of the type of evidence sought. Evidence can include a wide variety of resources, to include:

- empirical, primary journal articles located via traditional databases;
- graded, hierarchical resources discoverable via specialized databases that organize results by specific evidence levels; and
- local resources that provide guidance on an issue such as hospital handbooks, policy and practice guides for a specific floor or unit, and the counsel of experienced colleagues.

Once a shared understanding has been reached regarding the type of evidence needed, librarians can more confidently proceed in offering research assistance.

Also unique to health sciences research are clinical point-of-care resources. Some traditional research databases offer point-of-care resources, such as patient care sheets and evidence summaries for providers. Clinicians can also benefit from databases that are more strictly clinical in nature and designed to help inform the course of treatment. Many of these databases integrate directly into patients' electronic health records and are powerful, easily accessible tools for health care practitioners.

EMPLOY EFFECTIVE SEARCH STRATEGIES

Once researchers have selected the databases in which they will perform their searches, they are wise to familiarize themselves with the limits that are available to them within each data set. A good approach for librarians teaching patrons how to utilize databases is to describe the limits as options or strategies. There are no right or wrong searches or limit combinations, but it's important that they know what each selected limit will do. Teaching patrons the differences, benefits, and drawbacks of each limit is an important part of equipping them with the autonomy to use databases efficiently.

Evidence-based practice and clinical databases offer highly specialized limits. Researchers can effortlessly limit to specific genres of evidence in EBP databases. Point-of-care databases offer clinicians limits related to symptoms, coexisting conditions, patient population, and more.

Equally beneficial is teaching patrons how limits are designed to work. Although most databases now seamlessly create Boolean searches on behalf of the researcher, the researcher benefits from understanding the nuances between limiting options that combine search results or exclude items from results.

UTILIZE CONTROLLED VOCABULARY

Every discipline will have its own jargon. Experts in the field will use it comfortably, but those new to a discipline will have to become acquainted with the terminology used within their chosen field of study. For the researcher, learning this terminology can enhance their search strategies and refine their results. This is most certainly true when working with health sciences databases, as many of them are built upon a specific controlled vocabulary: MeSH terminology. Established by the National Library of Medicine and regularly updated to incorporate new terminology and modes of describing health sciences issues, the acronym MeSH stands for "medical subject headings." Many databases, to include numerous licensed health sciences databases and open access databases such as PubMed, are built upon MeSH vocabulary.

A way to introduce the concept of controlled vocabulary to novice researchers is to explain that there may be many terms to describe a situation or condition. These terms may be interchangeable, but by unlocking the terminology used in a specific database, they will maximize their search efficiency. For example, the terms *tumor* and *malignancy*, as well as names of specific cancer types, may all be used to describe the same thing. A particular term may not be more "correct" or "better" than the others, but of the options, there is likely one that will unlock the most relevant results for the researcher. When the researcher finds an article that is a good fit, taking a look at the subject terms that have been assigned to it within the database will generally provide leads to similar results within that database.

Formatting searches around controlled vocabulary works for most discipline databases. The practice of doing this over time allows the researcher to develop a cache of highly specific, effective search terms on which they can rely when they have an information need. An initiative that health sciences researchers can undertake to prepare themselves for future research is to spend time exploring the MeSH database, which will allow them to become more familiar with the MeSH tree structure, the trunk, and its branches. This familiarity will lead to insight on terminology and hierarchical relationships within their specialty. To learn more about MeSH, visit the MeSH tutorial: https://www.nlm.nih.gov/bsd/disted/meshtutorial/themeshdatabase/.

ANALYZE SEARCH RESULTS AND MODIFY SUBSEQUENT SEARCHES

The proficiencies listed up to this point have largely focused on preparing to research. Mastery of each of the above steps can lead to a highly refined results set. However, the experienced researcher understands that, at this point, the hard work is not completed but, rather, about to begin. The final limit that must be added to every potential supporting article cannot be performed by the database: it must be applied by the researcher in the form of close analysis of the refined results list.

Whereas novice undergraduates might be tempted to simply pick the top three results on the first page, upper-graduates and beyond will recognize the need for carefully selected articles that closely match their information need. Researchers can analyze each result quickly via initial assessment and then more in depth after determining that it might be a good fit for their research. The title will give the first indication, as will the genre of the result listed. Citation information can yield quick results—much can be learned from the name of the journal in which the article appeared, the date of publication, and the page range (length) of the article. For example, a one-page resource in a scholarly journal will generally not comprise a full research study.

Next, the subject terms can point to the finer points of the article and determine relevance. Per our earlier discussions of MeSH terminology, the researcher familiar with the nuances of terminology within their discipline can fully leverage the subjects listed for an article and quickly assess the article's fit. As a final means of evaluating an article for fit, the abstract will provide a clear snapshot of what lies inside the full text of the article. After a relatively quick evaluation of a given article based on the above elements, the researcher can feel confident about investing the time to read the full article and determine if there are any points for incorporation into their own research.

An article has value beyond what it can offer in and of itself. The researcher can take an article that's a good fit and 1) investigate citations that informed it by utilizing the works cited page and 2) investigate articles that their good-fit article informed by looking at who subsequently cited it. There are licensed resources that assist with this process, but a powerful open access resource accessible freely to all is Google Scholar and its "Cited By" link for each article in the database (take a look at https://scholar.google.com/).

At times, a researcher will not be satisfied with the results that they receive. The temptation is to become frustrated and decide that their topic is "bad" or simply not discussed in the literature. On occasion, this might actually be the case. But generally, spending time reexamining the research question, the databases selected, and the search strategies used will lead to "aha" moments that can help them uncover the literature they are seeking.

EXPLORATION IN ACTION: CASE STUDIES

Mapping the Information Literacy Skill Sets and Professional Standards of Upper-Division Nursing Students onto a Collectively Developed Rubric

Contributors: Katelyn Angell, MLIS, MA (Associate Professor and Coordinator of Library Instruction, LIU Brooklyn Library, Long Island University, Brooklyn Campus); and Gloria Willson, MLIS, MPH (Assistant Director, Programs, the Knowledge Center at the Augustus C. Long Health Sciences Library, Columbia University Irving Medical Center)

Frame—Searching as Strategic Exploration. Students develop the competencies to search and find quality, reliable health information resources for their growth as nursing professionals and to provide evidence-based care. All five other frames are associated with the project.

Target Audience: Librarians and instructors of undergraduate nursing programs. The lesson may also be adapted to other health sciences disciplines.

Setting: To be used with undergraduate nursing students in conjunction with nursing faculty to assess information literacy skills in research papers, particularly PICO assignments. Nursing faculty can bring courses with a major research paper component to the library. The faculty member and librarian can meet with each student individually and use the rubric to provide real-time feedback. Performance indicators from library and nursing core professional documents can help students flourish as future nursing professionals and information-literate citizens.

Learning Outcomes

For Librarians:

1. Librarians can learn how the ACRL Framework, when mapped to professional standards of practice, can be used to discover where information literacy skills are essential to mastering select professional competencies/skills.
2. Librarians can gain new ideas for tools to provide to teaching faculty to enhance their own outcome assessment efforts.

For Students:

1. Undergraduate nursing students will be provided with evaluation feedback that maps their information literacy skills to integral competencies of their future profession.

Exploration at a Glance: Quick Tips for Busy Librarians

Searching as Strategic Exploration

Searching for information is often nonlinear and iterative, requiring the evaluation of a range of information sources and the mental flexibility to pursue alternate avenues as new understanding develops.

http://www.ala.org/acrl/standards/ilframework

Q: What is searching?
A: Using carefully crafted strategies to locate information.

Characteristics of Searching:

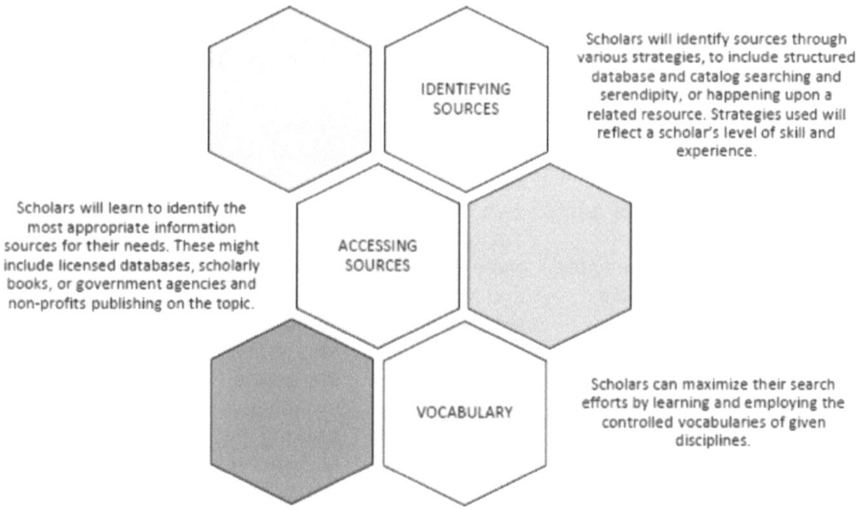

Special considerations for the health sciences:

- ❑ Health sciences literature is often located in discipline-specific databases. In the absence of a federated search tool, scholars should take care to consider relevant databases of aligned disciplines that might be able to inform their topic.
- ❑ Numerous health sciences databases are built upon the National Library of Medicine's MeSH terminology. Learning MeSH tree structures will lead to precise, efficient searches for scholars.
- ❑ Non-MeSH databases will provide subject headings that will lead scholars to the preferred vocabulary employed by the database.

2. Students will benefit from their research papers being assessed by both nursing and library faculty.

Assessment: A formal assessment method has not yet been developed.

Activity: The rubric (table 7.1) is used to evaluate nursing research papers for critical information competencies outlined in the American Nurses Association Standards of Professional Nursing Practice and the ACRL Framework. Both student scores and interrater reliability of the investigators can be calculated and reported. Optimal application entails evaluation of student artifacts by both library and nursing faculty.

Reference: Willson, G., & Angell, K. (2017). Mapping the Association of College and Research Libraries information literacy framework and nursing professional standards onto an assessment rubric. *Journal of the Medical Library Association, 105*(2), 150–154. doi:https://doi.org/10.5195/jmla.2017.39

Table 7.1. Information Literacy and Nursing Professional Standards Assessment Rubric

ACRL Frame	ANA Standard	Beginning (1)	Developing (2)	Exemplary (3)
Authority Is Constructed and Contextual	5D (Prescribes evidence-based treatments, therapies, and procedures considering the health care consumers' comprehensive health care needs)	Seldom acknowledges development of own authoritative voice in nursing and seldom recognizes the responsibilities this entails, including seeking accuracy and reliability, respecting intellectual property, and participating in community of practice	Partially acknowledges development of own authoritative voice in nursing and partially recognizes the responsibilities this entails, including seeking accuracy and reliability, respecting intellectual property, and participating in community of practice	Fully acknowledges development of own authoritative voice in nursing and fully recognizes the responsibilities this entails, including seeking accuracy and reliability, respecting intellectual property, and participating in community of practice
Information Creation as a Process	9 (Participates, as appropriate to education level and position, in the formulation of evidence-based practice through research)	Seldom develops, in their own creation process, an understanding that their choices impact the purposes for which their information product will be	Partially develops, in their own creation process, an understanding that their choices impact the purposes for which their information product will be	Fully develops, in their own creation process, an understanding that their choices impact the purposes for which their information product will be used and the

		used and the message it conveys	used and the message it conveys	message it conveys
Information Has Value	4 (Integrates current scientific evidence, trends, and research)	Seldom gives credit to the original ideas of others through proper attribution and citation	Partially gives credit to the original ideas of others through proper attribution and citation	Fully gives credit to the original ideas of others through proper attribution and citation
Research as Inquiry	1 (Synthesizes available data, information, and knowledge relevant to the situation to identify patterns and variables)	Seldom draws reasonable conclusions based on the analysis and interpretation of information	Partially draws reasonable conclusions based on the analysis and interpretation of information	Fully draws reasonable conclusions based on the analysis and interpretation of information
Scholarship as Conversatio n	5 (Applies appropriate knowledge of major health problems and cultural diversity in implementing the plan of care)	Seldom identifies the contribution that the selected articles make to disciplinary knowledge	Partially identifies the contribution that the selected articles make to disciplinary knowledge	Fully identifies the contribution that the selected articles make to disciplinary knowledge
Searching as Strategic Exploration	3 (Considers associated risks, benefits, costs, current scientific evidence, expected trajectory of the condition, and clinical expertise when formulating expected outcomes)	Seldom determines the initial scope of the assignment required to meet their information needs	Partially determines the initial scope of the assignment required to meet their information needs	Fully determines the initial scope of the assignment required to meet their information needs

Source: Courtesy of Katelyn Angell and Gloria Willson.

Finding, Interpreting, and Communicating Scientific Information

Contributor: Andrea C. Kepsel, MLIS, AHIP (Health Sciences Educational Technology Librarian, Michigan State University Libraries

Frame—Searching as Strategic Exploration. Students are provided with a search topic and asked to search both health sciences databases and websites.

They are asked to compare the results and identify which they would use when communicating with either colleagues or clients.

Other associated frames: Authority Is Constructed and Contextual.

Target Audience: Undergraduate veterinary technology (LVT) students. The lesson may also be adapted to other health sciences disciplines such as nursing or medicine.

Setting: To be used in a two-part in-person instruction series with undergraduate veterinary technology students enrolled in a hospital communications and procedures course. Students in the course are developing professional and client communication skills.

Learning Outcomes: Students will identify reliable places to search when looking for information to answer a clinical question. Students will judge the appropriateness of the resource depending on the audience and describe why it was selected.

Assessment: Formative assessment is built into the Searching the Resources Exercise reflection questions. Additionally, at the end of the instruction series students are asked to write a one-minute paper on the most important thing they learned and what is still unclear.

Activity: The Searching the Resources Exercise will provide students with an opportunity to explore different resources and compare the types of information found. The exercise can be completed individually or in groups in class. Some knowledge on forming a good search strategy is necessary, whether from a previous activity or lecture. Resources used can be modified based on availability or discipline.

Searching the Resources Exercise: Your client's dog has recently been diagnosed with diabetes and is trying to understand the relationship between diet, exercise, and insulin production. You have been asked to find information for the client, as well as research that can be used to educate the care team on diabetes management.

Search Strategy

1. List the keywords you will use in your search. Remember to include any synonyms or alternate keywords.
2. Write down your search strategy, including search connectors, truncation, or quotation marks, *exactly* how you will enter it into a search box.
3. List any limits or filters you will apply to narrow down your search results.

Now that you have decided on your search strategy, try it out in three different resources: CAB Abstracts, PubMed, and Veterinary Partner. Answer the accompanying questions and select one result for each resource.

Search #1: CAB Abstracts

1. How many results did your search strategy produce?
2. What limits or filters did you use?
3. Did you need to modify your search and try again? If so, what was your new search strategy, and how many results did it produce?

Select one item from your search results you think can be used to answer the clinical question and record its citation:

1. Why did you select this item?
2. How do you know it provides reliable information?

Search #2: PubMed

1. How many results did your search strategy produce?
2. What limits or filters did you use?
3. Did you need to modify your search and try again? If so, what was your new search strategy, and how many results did it produce?

Select one item from your search results you think can be used to answer the clinical question and record its citation:

1. Why did you select this item?
2. How do you know it provides reliable information?

Search #3: Veterinary Partner (https://veterinarypartner.vin.com)

1. How many results did your search strategy produce?
2. What limits or filters did you use?
3. Did you need to modify your search and try again? If so, what was your new search strategy, and how many results did it produce?

Select one item from your search results you think can be used to answer the clinical question and record its citation:

1. Why did you select this item?
2. How do you know it provides reliable information?

Reflection Questions

1. What resource do you think is the best to search when looking for information for your client? For members of your care team? Explain why.
2. Did your original search strategy give you enough results to review? Too many? Too few? Did it work better or worse in one resource compared to the others?
3. Did any of your search results provide you with new keywords to try that you had not thought of initially? What were they?
4. If you could try the searches again, what changes would you make to your search strategy? Why do you think this will work better?
5. Are there other resources beyond the three used in this exercise that you think you should search? What are they, and why do you want to use them?

Exploring Popular Sources and Published Research in Food Science

Contributor: Lea Leininger, MLIS (Health Sciences Librarian, Jackson Library, UNC Greensboro)

Frame—Searching as Strategic Exploration. Students suggest sources for topic ideas through Poll Everywhere or a similar tool. Students are encouraged to look at various sources for topic ideas—published recipes, websites with recipe reviews, and food science journals. Students are shown a food science journal and discuss language used in a research article. Students generate keywords and search a database such as ScienceDirect or SpringerLink for food science articles.

Other associated frames: Research as Inquiry, Authority Is Constructed and Contextual.

Target Audience: Undergraduate and graduate students in a food science research lab course. The lesson can be adapted for non-lab courses that have an assignment that begins with topic selection.

Setting: One-shot library instruction for food science students beginning a semester-long project. This lesson plan can be used in a computer lab or in a classroom with laptops/other devices and internet access. The lesson plan can be adapted for virtual instruction.

Students begin topic exploration. They will need multiple information sources to support the creation and testing of several versions of a food product. A successful project proposal will include a food science research article, but the instructor and the librarian understand that students might need additional time after one library instruction session to compare topic ideas and explore sources. The library instruction is intended to guide students in exploring information sources to support research projects, while the instructor is present to answer questions about lab resources and project feasibility.

Learning Outcomes: Students will explore a variety of information resources to support a food science research project. Students will generate topic ideas, keywords, and practice article searching.

Assessment

Part 1. End-of-Session Google Poll: Students will answer the following questions:

1. Where have you gone for topic and keyword ideas? _ Recipe website _ Food science journal _ Friend/classmate _ Instructor _ Librarian
2. Which topic are you interested in researching?
3. Which keywords have you tried?
4. Has your topic changed since searching and discussing your ideas?
5. Do you have any questions for the librarian at this point?

Part 2. End-of-Semester Reference List Evaluation: Students will identify a food science research article and additional sources to support the project.

- Excellent—Multiple primary research articles focusing on food science: a preparation technique, substitution, analysis of food components, or similar. Several other sources also used, for instance, review articles, food science websites and/or texts, websites or other sources for the general public. Other sources might address health effects of foods or special dietary needs of a specific condition/population.
- Acceptable—At least one primary research article focusing on food science: a preparation technique, substitution, analysis of food components, or similar. At least one other source cited: review article, food science websites and/or text, and a source intended for the general public. Other sources might address health effects of foods or special dietary needs of a specific condition/population.
- Needs improvement—No primary research article in food science.

Activity—Exploring Topics

1. Have students respond to an online poll asking where they like to go for recipe and substitution ideas. Show the results and discuss.
2. Browse a journal such as *LWT-Food Science and Technology* that has examples of research articles on different topics.
3. Encourage students to look at different sources while they come up with three topic ideas.

- Not sure where to start? Browsing a food science journal = inspiration + a source for your references list.
- Like an ingredient/recipe, but not sure what to test? Do a Google search such as *brownie substitution* or search a website like epicurious.com and check reviews for additions or substitutions.
- Recipes/techniques that I would like to test:

Research Article: Looking at a research article, discuss hallmarks of a primary report of research, for instance, a description of how the authors gathered their own data.

Keywords and Searching: Discuss language that you see in a journal article versus language in other sources. Encourage students to help brainstorm different ways to describe a food or recipe (create a mind map on a whiteboard). Encourage students to write useful terms that they have seen for their own topic (table 7.2).

Model an article search, reminding students to use *and* when they want to search more than one keyword at a time.

Investigating Public Health Indexes

Contributor: Xan Goodman (Health Sciences Librarian, Associate Professor, University Libraries, University of Nevada, Las Vegas)

Frames—Search as Strategic Exploration and *Authority Is Constructed and Contextual.* Students are challenged to use the frames Search as Strategic Exploration and Authority Is Constructed and Contextual to explore databases and indexes relevant to their final research assignment. There is overlap between these two frames because as students contemplate strategic searching they must also consider the authority of the resources they gather for their final paper.

Target Audience: Graduate and undergraduate public health students.

Setting: This information literacy lesson is to be used with undergraduate or graduate public health students in preparation for a research-intensive paper. The lesson can be used virtually or in the classroom. The time allotted for instruction is 75 minutes.

Table 7.2. Recipe Brainstorming Exercise

Food/Recipe Idea	Substitution or Other Variable to Test	Properties to Investigate
		taste, texture, acceptability, sensory, quality, characteristics

Learning Outcomes

1. Students will locate scientific public health literature relevant to the course content.
2. Students will develop an ability to explain what a relevant public health source is for their assignment.
3. Students will describe the differences between indexes and which to choose and for what purpose.

Assessment

A formative in-class assessment is completed with two questions:

1. What is the most important thing you learned in today's library workshop?
2. And what remains unclear? Questions get at the muddiest point for learners from the lesson.

Preparation

Prepare a PowerPoint presentation, a muddiest point assessment in print or electronically, and a library worksheet. Optionally, create a course LibGuide with curated paid library databases and indexes and freely available indexes. Here are a few examples of paid library public health indexes or databases: GreenFILE, ScienceDirect, BioOne Complete, and Agriculture & Environmental Science Database. Here are a few examples of freely available indexes: AGRICOLA, Directory of Open Access Journals (DOAJ), and BioMed Central including the internet search engine Google Scholar. Select article examples of scholarly and non-scholarly articles for the worksheet activity.

Prior to implementing this lesson the librarian meets with the instructor to determine how to infuse information literacy into the course. The librarian creates an instruction plan table with five elements: a learning outcome, a frame, knowledge practices, dispositions, and outcomes to show evidence of learning (table 7.3).

Lesson Plan

The librarian explains the purpose, tasks, and learning criteria to students:

> The purpose of this lesson is to guide your critical thinking to locate and determine authority of sources selected for a final paper. You will identify at least three indexes or databases and be able to describe differences between indexes. You will also explain hallmarks of legitimate public health sources. We will complete the following tasks: two activities and viewing a video. By the end of this lesson, you will demonstrate success if you experience an

Table 7.3. Instruction Plan

Learning Outcome	Frame	Knowledge Practice	Disposition	Evidence of Learning
Locate scientific public health literature	Searching as strategic exploration	Determine the scope of the question or task required to meet one's needs	Show through their searching that they value persistence, adaptability, and flexibility; understand that first attempts at searching don't always pay off; and are willing to analyze needs at the beginning of information searches	Able to identify and critically analyze sources for inclusion in the final project
Explain how they determine what a legitimate public health source might be	Authority is constructed and contextual	Identify markers of authority when engaging with information, understanding the elements that might temper authority	Aware of the importance of assessing content critically to the best of their ability	Describe hallmarks of scientific and lay public health literature
Know the differences between indexes and which to choose and for what purpose	Searching as strategic exploration	Demonstrate the importance of matching information needs and search strategies to appropriate search tools	Show through their searching that they value persistence, adaptability, and flexibility	Can name at least three indexes or database tools they use to search and describe how they use those tools

increase in confidence with your ability to locate scientific public health literature.

Instruction Session

The librarian divides the class into groups (groups of three or four are acceptable). Distribute an article and a library worksheet to each group. Explain that each group will select a spokesperson and a recorder. The recorder will list three reasons why the group article is either a scientific or lay article or list three reasons why their article is not a scientific or lay article. Give groups time to discuss among themselves. The librarian will circulate around the room as groups discuss to listen and answer questions. The spokesperson from each group will come to the front of the class to explain how their groups determined if an article is a scientific or lay article.

The format of this lesson allows students to jump right into assessing an article and gives the librarian a chance to observe how students are evaluating articles. The librarian can build on students' critical thinking skills using the frame Authority Is Constructed and Contextual. The librarian will guide the discussion to highlight hallmarks of a scientific and lay literature. Some hallmarks of scientific literature students will point out might include references, authors with advanced degrees, and the presence of charts, figures, or tables. Alternatively, hallmarks of lay literature might consist of an author who is a journalist, an article from a popular publication, or lack of references. Each point allows for open discussion between the students and librarian about critically assessing an article. Transition to a discussion about how to search for literature. Have students view the following video tutorial: "Finding Articles" (https://vimeo.com/179489136). This tutorial is freely available on Vimeo.

After reviewing the video, prompt the students to write down three indexes or databases they have used in their own personal searching. Next have them select one of those databases and write why that resource is a relevant resource for their assignment. In their groups, have a person from each group report about why they chose an index or database. The librarian will write the name of the index or database in a blank slide in the PowerPoint presentation and add differences about each index or database for discussion. This exercise is valuable for students because they learn from their colleagues about indexes and databases to locate scholarly literature. Rather than have each student search a database or index, we discuss as a class their rationale for selecting a particular database or index and why that resource is an excellent choice for their topic. This allows the librarian to share expertise about why specific databases or indexes might be more or less helpful, and it uncovers and exposes the searching habits of upper-level undergraduate and graduate students. The librarian will learn what students have been doing. If the librarian has created a course LibGuide before the instruction session, students can be directed to a guide of curated resources composed of paid library databases and indexes as well as open indexes on the internet like the Directory of Open Access Journals (DOAJ).

This lesson opens up channels for fruitful discussion between the librarian as expert information professional and students. As the lesson comes to closure, have the students answer in two or three sentences their understanding of the concepts of Searching as Strategic Exploration and Authority Is

Constructed and Contextual. Leave time for discussion about the two frames to answer any questions students might have about the frames and how they relate to their project. Students might ask how to strategically determine their information need to select the best indexes or databases for their project. Finally, ask students to complete the muddiest point questions. As a follow-up to the muddiest point assessment, the librarian will answer unclear questions on the course LibGuide.

Library Worksheet

1. List at least three reasons why your article *is* a scientific or lay article.
2. List at least three reasons why your article is *not* a scientific or lay article.
3. List the names of three indexes/databases you have previously used.
4. Select one index/database and explain in two or three sentences why this is a relevant source to locate scientific literature for your assignment.
5. Write two or three sentences to explain your understanding of:

    a. Searching as Strategic Exploration.
    b. Authority Is Constructed and Contextual.

Muddiest Point Assessment

1. What is the most important thing you learned in today's library workshop?
2. What remains unclear?

Searching for Information in Communication Disorders

Contributor: Adelia Grabowsky, MLIS (Health Sciences Librarian, Ralph Draughon Library, Auburn University

Frame—Searching as Strategic Exploration. Students will develop and refine search strategies for two health sciences databases using both convergent and divergent thinking as well as different types of searching language. Students will also manage their search results. Other associated frames: Research as Inquiry.

Target Audience: Graduate communication disorders students (speech-language pathology MS and MCD; audiology, AuD). The lesson may also be adapted to other health sciences disciplines, including graduate nursing students.

Setting: To be used with students in a research methods class that requires students to develop a research proposal over the course of the semester.

Students are required to search the professional literature to determine where gaps exist in order to develop a feasible proposal.

Learning Outcomes: Students will use different types of searching language (keywords, subject headings) to design a search and refine the search based on results. Students will explore two sources of information, understanding how those resources are organized in order to better access relevant information. Students will practice saving results and finding full text of results.

Assessment

Formative: An in-class quiz (using clickers) to test students' knowledge of Boolean operators.

Summative: Pre- and post-questions about a prior information-seeking frustration. Before class, students are asked to list the biggest problem/frustration encountered the last time they searched for information for a paper/project. After class, students are asked if they learned something that would help with their previous problem. If they answer *yes* or *maybe*, they are asked to briefly describe what they learned that would help. Pre- and post-answers are matched up, coded, and analyzed to determine if students were able to describe an appropriate solution to their stated problem.

Class Outline

For this class, the two sources of information explored were PubMed and PsycINFO, but databases can be changed based on target audience and available resources. Class time is 1 hour and 15 minutes and consists of alternating librarian demo/student practice as follows:

- The librarian introduces subject guide and asks students to answer pre-assessment question (~3 minutes).
- The librarian introduces core databases for communication disorders (~2 minutes).
- The librarian introduces a sample topic (Treatment options for children with apraxia of speech) then leads students in selecting major concepts for searching. Students use the in-class worksheet to write down their own topic (or choose one of the provided topics), then repeat selecting major concepts for their topic (~5 minutes).
- The librarian introduces the concept of synonyms/related terms, asks students to help brainstorm synonyms/related terms for each concept in the sample topic. Students repeat the brainstorming of synonyms/related terms for their own topics (~5 minutes).
- A short three-question quiz (PowerPoint and clickers) tests students' knowledge of how to use *and* and *or* to combine concepts and synonyms.

Typically, there are some wrong answers for each question. In the ensuing discussion, Venn diagrams are used to illustrate the use of *and* and *or* (~5 minutes).

- The librarian introduces PsycINFO and demonstrates searching using sample topic, including how to use *or* to connect synonyms, how to use limits, and how to view abstracts to determine the effectiveness of the search. After a short discussion of what subject headings are, the librarian demonstrates how to find subject headings in the results list and how to add articles to the folder to save them. Students repeat searching in PsycINFO with their topics, saving relevant articles to the folder (~18 minutes).
- The librarian demonstrates how to e-mail results from the folder; students repeat with the articles they found (~5 minutes).
- The librarian introduces PubMed and demonstrates searching with a single search box and how to use the MeSH database to find subject headings. Students use the MeSH database to find subject headings for their concepts and record them on the worksheet (~5 minutes).
- In PubMed, the librarian demonstrates using limits, viewing abstracts, and saving searches to the clipboard. Students repeat, searching PubMed with their topics (~15 minutes).
- The librarian demonstrates how to find full text, including how to make interlibrary loan requests. Students try finding full text for an article they saved (~5 minutes).
- To wrap up, the librarian shows subject guide and asks students to answer post-assessment question. (~2 minutes)

Activity—In-Class Worksheet

(Note: sample topics are provided because library instruction takes place early in the semester and students do not always have a topic in mind. Sample topics can be adjusted based on target audience.)

Write down your own topic *or* choose one of the sample topics listed below:

- Tense use to diagnose language impairment in children
- Use of telehealth to diagnose dysphagia
- Interventions to improve swallowing in preterm infants
- Assessing language development in children with autism

Topic:

1. Circle main concepts in topic.

2. List synonyms/related terms to try for each concept:
3. Look for a subject heading for each concept and list it here:

Failing Forward: Strategic Searching for Physician Assistants

Contributor: Allison Papini, MLIS (Research & Instruction Librarian, Adjunct Clinical Assistant Professor, Douglas and Judith Krupp Library, Bryant University)

Frame—Searching as Strategic Exploration. Learners are often intellectually curious but lack the time and/or skills needed to move beyond initial search results. This exercise will provide them with the tools they need to become effective researchers.

Other associated frames: Authority Is Constructed and Contextual and Information Creation as a Process.

Target Audience: Graduate physician assistant (MPAS). The lesson may also be adapted to health sciences classes at the graduate and undergraduate level, depending on program and student prior knowledge.

Setting: This session is the first step in a research project that will run for the duration of the course. This course is taught by a research and instruction librarian face-to-face in a Team-Based Learning (TBL) (Michaelsen & Sweet, 2011, 41–51) seminar-style classroom. The lesson may be adapted for virtual learners. This is intended to be a 3-hour class session, though it can be divided into a series of classes as needed.

Learning Outcomes: By the end of this session, students will be able to:

1. formulate a research question that reflects the tenets of evidence-based medicine, using PICO(T) as framework in order to develop a search strategy; and
2. experiment with a variety of resources, including grey literature, in order to acquire sources that satisfy the information need for the assignment.

Assessment: Students will be evaluated at the start of the session using TBL readiness assessments (individual and team) to check for understanding of the material posted on Blackboard. These readiness assessments are brief multiple-choice quizzes of 5–10 questions that will be completed as an individual and then repeated as part of a team. Students will document their use of PICOT(T) (Medical University of South Carolina, 2018) in order to generate a foreground question and different iterations of their search strategy. Students will be graded on the quality of their search strategy as well as how they adapted the strategy to find the best resources. This session is intended to help the students start the research that they will use for a final team research presentation that will be the major assessment for the course.

Activity—Before Class

Students will be required to watch a video reviewing the resources they will be focusing on during the class session—PubMed, UpToDate, Clinical Key, and Cochrane Library. The students will also learn how to access the individual resources and how to use the search features in each. The video and supporting materials will be posted to Blackboard and available to students 3 days before the class session.

Teams will be asked to come prepared with two topics they are interested in investigating. The diseases/conditions they will be researching will be ones commonly seen by clinicians, including diabetes, obesity-related issues, and heart disease.

Activity—In-Class PICOT(T) Exercise

Using the topic you have selected with your team, brainstorm elements to outline the following:

- Patient / Population / Problem
- Intervention
- Comparison
- Outcome
- Type of Question
- Type of Article

In the next step, you will incorporate the terms you generated in the PICOT(T) outline to complete your search strategy.

Activity—Search Strategy Exercise

1. Topic:
2. Area of focus:
3. Circle the types of resources needed (books, journal articles, reviews, grey literature):

    - Journal articles
    - Reviews
    - Books
    - Grey literature
    - Other ____________

4. Circle the highest level or levels of evidence appropriate for the type of question (Duke University Medical Center Archives, 2018). Be

open to different levels of evidence—you'll be able to narrow the results later.

- Meta-analysis
- Systematic review
- Randomized controlled trial
- Cohort study
- Case control study
- Case series / case report
- Other reviews of the literature
- Clinical reference texts

5. Keywords:
6. Synonyms / alternate spellings:
7. MeSH subject headings:
8. Broader terms:
9. Narrower terms:
10. Team notes on results: What was successful? What needed to be adjusted in order to locate the best available evidence? Be sure to document these during and after each search.

Students will repeat the search at least twice more in class, incorporating and documenting the changes they have made to resources, keywords, and other necessary adjustments. By the end of this session, students will be able to move beyond doing a single search, instead demonstrating creativity and mental flexibility. Students will come away with the tools to create and refine searches in order to gather the best-level evidence and highest-quality results for their research and ultimately clinical practice.

References

Duke University Medical Center Archives. (2018). Evidence-based practice: Study design. Retrieved from https://guides.mclibrary.duke.edu/ebm/studydesign

Medical University of South Carolina. (2018). Evidence-based dentistry: PICOTT. Retrieved from https://musc.libguides.com/ebd/PICOTT

Michaelsen, L. K., & Sweet, M. (2011). Team-based learning. *New Directions for Teaching & Learning, 2011*(128), 41–51. Retrieved from https://doi.org/10.1002/tl.467

All the Right Moves: How PubMed Articulates Your Search Terms

Contributor: Heather A. Johnson, MLIS (Research and Education Librarian, Biomedical Libraries, Dartmouth College)

Frame—Searching as Strategic Exploration

Target Audience: This lesson plan is designed for graduate occupational and physical therapy students.

Discipline: This lesson plan was originally developed for a surgical residency in otolaryngology. I have adapted it for several specialties, including occupational and physical therapy. The proposed lesson plan is for physical/occupational therapy students and professionals. The lesson will include suggestions for modifying for other specialties.

Setting: The proposed lesson was developed for physical and occupational therapists and assistants. The purpose of the session was to show postgraduate professionals how to search the peer-reviewed literature for the purpose of supporting research or clinical care. However, this lesson could be taught without modification in an academic setting for the purpose of preparing students to write a research paper.

Learning Outcomes: At the end of the session, students should be able to:

1. explain the difference between a MeSH term and keyword,
2. define the MeSH hierarchy, and
3. translate keywords to MeSH terms using the MeSH database in PubMed.

Activity: This lesson plan is designed to introduce students and postgraduate professionals to the MeSH database in PubMed. During this 1-hour session, students learn the basics of constructing keyword searches using Boolean operators (e.g., tennis elbow *or* lateral epicondylitis) and employing the MeSH database to construct focused searches. The 1-hour session includes a 20-minute overview of how to create keyword searches and how to use the MeSH database. During the last 40 minutes, students work in pairs to "translate" their keywords to MeSH terms and create search strategies using a combination of MeSH terms and subheadings.

Finding the Evidence to Support a Nursing Evidence-Based Project

Contributors: Brenda Fay, MLIS (Librarian Specialist, Advocate Aurora Library Network, Aurora Health Care Wisconsin); Kathy Koch, MLIS (Librarian, Advocate Aurora Library Network, Aurora Health Care Wisconsin); and Rita Mitchell, MM, MLIS (Lead Librarian, Advocate Aurora Library Network, Aurora Health Care Wisconsin)

Frame—Searching as Strategic Exploration. Nurses are challenged to formulate a question, develop keywords, select appropriate evidence-based resources, and critically evaluate citations and abstracts. Other associated frames: Research as Inquiry.

Target Audience: Professional nurses. The lesson may also be adapted to other health sciences disciplines, including student nurses and other student or practicing allied health professionals.

Setting: To be used with new RN graduates in a hospital-based nurse residency program preparing to research the literature regarding a clinical situation they want to improve on their unit. This was developed for large groups in a conference room setting.

Learning Outcomes: Professional nurses will be able to formulate a research question, develop and refine search strategies, and evaluate retrieved clinical literature.

Assessment

Formative: In-session, low-stakes group work.

- Question generating group activity
- Keyword brainstorming

Formative: In-session, strategic-questioning group work.

- Defining relevant clinical literature discussion

Summative/Final Product

- Nursing evidence-based project completion

Activities: Completed as a one-time session in a large group setting with multiple cohorts across the health care system.

Develop a Question Activity (10 Minutes)

1. Take a clinical scenario and demonstrate to the students how to translate that into a question(s).
2. Distribute a different scenario to use with small groups or partner.
3. Give groups 5 minutes to generate a question from the scenario.
4. Ask for volunteers to read the question(s) they generated.

Scenario 1: You're a nurse working on a med-surg floor, and you notice that the telemetry patches are not being changed every 24 hours. You want to find out if there are any best practices for this and if not changing them often enough can contribute to skin issues.

Possible keywords:

- Electrode
- EKC / ECG
- Telemetry

- Electrocardiography
- Skin safety, skin injury, skin care
- Daily, frequently, frequency, 24 hours

Scenario 2: Your unit is getting low HCAHPS scores for noise levels, and you want to start a project to help patients get better sleep and reduce the amount of noise at night. You're wondering what other hospitals have had success with.

Possible keywords:

- Quiet, quiet at night
- Noise control or reduction
- Better or improved sleep
- Sleep, sleep hygiene, sleep promotion
- Sleep problems, insomnia, sleep deprivation
- Hospital environment
- HCAHPS (Hospital Consumer Assessment of Healthcare Providers and Systems)
- Patient satisfaction
- Earplugs
- Sleep masks
- Relaxation
- Lavender essential oil

Scenario 3: You are a nurse attempting to improve processes when patients are admitted onto the med-surg floors from the Emergency Department. Important information is missing such as meds, mental status, how they move, and what protocols or assessments have been done. How can you improve this intake process on your unit?

Possible keywords:

- Handoff, hand-over, report
- Inpatient unit, medical surgical unit/ward
- Emergency department
- Transfer
- Communication
- Outcomes
- Adverse events
- Tool, model

Brainstorm Keywords Activity (5 Minutes)

1. Using the scenario from the previous activity, ask nurses to think about keywords.
2. Use word cloud / polling software for electronic responses (Poll Everywhere, SurveyPlanet). Alternatively, have markers at each table and invite nurses to write keywords on a whiteboard.

Explore Search Strategies Activity (15 Minutes)

1. The librarian will demonstrate a search using keywords generated by nurses.
2. Show advanced searching with keywords in at least two resources.
3. Discuss ways to filter results (date, age, gender).
4. Point out elements of search results to think critically about

    a. Date of publication—is it current?
    b. Type of article—is this original research, a review or summary, a conference abstract?
    c. Country of study or affiliation of author.
    d. Population characteristics—age, gender, hospital unit?

5. Demonstrate a search using different keywords.

Evaluate Search Results Activity (10 Minutes)

1. Before class, the librarian will perform a search on a scenario and pull three or four citations with abstracts for distribution in class. These will ideally be a mixture of criteria from #4 above (date, type of article, country of study, study population).
2. Have groups rank citations/abstracts.
3. Bring back to large group, share rankings, and discuss.

Index

About the Editors

Elizabeth G. Hinton, MSIS, AHIP, Rowland Medical Library, is instruction and research librarian and assistant professor at the University of Mississippi Medical Center's Rowland Medical Library, where she has been employed since 2012. After receiving her MS in information science from the University of Tennessee, Knoxville, she completed a postgraduate internship at the University of Tennessee Medical Center. In her current position, she is library liaison to the School of Nursing, where she holds a secondary faculty appointment and is a core faculty member of the Mississippi Centre for Evidence-Based Practice: A Joanna Briggs Institute Centre of Excellence and a trainer for the Joanna Briggs Institute Comprehensive Systematic Review Training Programme. Ms. Hinton is author or coauthor on several peer-reviewed journal articles and book chapters and has presented multiple posters and papers. She has also been the primary investigator on two grants for the improvement of library services.

Ms. Hinton is active in both the Medical Library Association and the southern chapter of the Medical Library Association. She is a senior member of AHIP, has been a member of the Rising Star Program leadership team, the MLA Credentialing Committee, and chair of the MLA Nursing and Allied Health Resources Section. Most notably, she received the MLA President's Award for her work on the MLA Education Steering Committee. She has also served SC/MLA as a member of the executive board and chair or member of several committees. Her professional interests include systematic reviews, library and educational assessment, and measuring scholarly output.

Lauren M. Young, MLIS, MA, AHIP, Harwell Goodwin Davis Library, is instruction coordinator for Reference and Research Services at Samford University's Davis Library and holds the rank of associate librarian. Her academic library career has seen equal time spent in technical services and public services roles, and she specializes in serving the information needs of health sciences programs and patrons. She enjoys institutional and library assessment work, having received training at the institutional and national levels.

In addition to her library work, Ms. Young was an instructor of English composition and literature courses for the Mississippi Virtual Community College for 10 years and remains active in and passionate about creating vivid online learning environments for distance learning students.

Ms. Young earned her MLIS from the University of Southern Mississippi and a BA and an MA in English from the University of Mississippi. She is an active member of state, regional, and national associations and a member of the Medical Library Association's Academy of Health Information Professionals at the distinguished level (AHIP-D). Her research interests include information and health literacy, interprofessional education, and Old English literary studies.

www.ingramcontent.com/pod-product-compliance
Ingram Content Group UK Ltd.
Pitfield, Milton Keynes, MK11 3LW, UK
UKHW012041150926
475560UK00001B/128

9 781538 11892